Titles in the **Contemporary Nursing Series**

- Nursing in Neurological Disorders
- Nursing of Children and Adolescents
- Advances in Cardiovascular Nursing
- The Nursing Process in Practice
- Nursing and the Aging Patient
- The Expanded Role of The Nurse
- Nursing and The Cancer Patient
- Human Sexuality: Nursing Implications
- Maternal and Newborn Care: Nursing Interventions
- The Dying Patient: A Nursing Perspective
- Nursing in Respiratory Diseases
- The Nurse in Community Mental Health
- Nursing in Cardiovascular Diseases
- Changing Patterns of Nursing Practice
- The Clinical Nurse Specialist

A compilation of articles selected
and reprinted from the **American Journal of Nursing,
Nursing Research,** and **Nursing Outlook**

Contemporary Nursing Series

NURSING IN NEUROLOGICAL DISORDERS

compiled by
Andrea B. O'Connor, R.N.

The American Journal of Nursing Company
New York

Copyright © 1976
The American Journal of Nursing Company
10 Columbus Circle
New York, New York 10019

All rights reserved. No part of this book, with the exception of brief excerpts for review, may be reproduced in any form or by any means without written permission from the publisher.

Library of Congress Catalog Number: 78-140949

Printed in the United States of America

FOREWORD

This present publication is the fifteenth book in the CONTEMPORARY NURSING SERIES. Launched in 1970 by the Educational Services Division of The American Journal of Nursing Company, the series has covered a wide range of subjects, ranging from such areas as nursing in cardiovascular and respiratory conditions to the broader issues of the expanded role of the nurse and the application of the nursing process to practice.

As readers of the series know, these paperback books are collections of selected articles in a particular subject area, all of the material having originally been published in one of The American Journal of Nursing Company's periodicals: the *American Journal of Nursing, Nursing Outlook, Nursing Research,* and *MCN The American Journal of Maternal Child Nursing.* The selection of articles for inclusion is not random. Instead, the magazines are carefully searched to identify the best and most appropriate material, the articles are subgrouped within each volume for the reader's convenience, and the final product is a compact reference source for the nurse who wishes to broaden or update her knowledge in a given subject area.

The response to the CONTEMPORARY NURSING SERIES has been both enthusiastic and gratifying. This encourages the Journal Company to believe that, through these books, it is continuing to expand its services to the nursing profession. In so doing, the Company is also accomplishing the goal established for it by its founders in 1900: "to present the most useful facts, the most progressive thought, and the latest news the profession has to offer in the most attractive form that can be secured."—PHILIP E. DAY, R.N., Publishing Director, The American Journal of Nursing Company.

PREFACE

This volume, the fifteenth book in the CONTEMPORARY NURSING SERIES, addresses the problems encountered in caring for persons with neurological and neuromuscular disorders. Due to the complexity of the nervous system, patients afflicted with such diseases present challenges to nurses working in acute or chronic care facilities or seeing clients in clinics or at home. Acute neurological disorders may involve any body system, requiring the nurse to remain alert for and intervene to prevent complications. During convalescence, rehabilitative measures are directed toward enabling the patient to attain his optimum level of function.

The articles in this volume were selected from the Journal Company's publications to represent a variety of neurological problems requiring nursing intervention for prevention, restoration of health, and rehabilitation. Most of the articles deal with the care of adults, but the information in them can be applied to the nursing of children and adolescents with similar disorders. While this book is by no means comprehensive, it does represent the latest thinking of experts across the country. As in the previous books in the CONTEMPORARY NURSING SERIES, the biographies accompanying the articles identify each author's background and position at the time the article was originally written and published.

Contents

SECTION I: Assessment and Diagnostic Testing

Assessing Station and Gait 1
    Mariah Snyder
    Rebecca Baum

Guidelines for the Care of Confused Patients 5
    Magdalena Morris
    Martha Rhodes

Optokinetic Nystagmus 12
    George L. Larsen

P.E.G. and Angiography: A Patient's Sensations 15
    Carol Ann Blackwell

Preparing a Patient for EEG 20
    Donald Shearer
    Betty Collins
    Donnell Creel

SECTION II: Some Common Neurological Disorders

Vascular and Tension Headaches 25
    Lois M. Hoskins

Epilepsy: A Controllable Disease 36
    Margaret Auld Bruya
    Rose Homan Bolin

Bringing Epilepsy Out of the Closet 55
    Laurale Harkness

Levodopa and Parkinsonism 59
    Marilyn Beaton Robinson

Improving Speech in Parkinson's Disease 71
    Elizabeth Erb

SECTION III: Disorders Requiring Neurosurgery or Acute Care

A Delicate Balance: Managing Airway Obstruction in
a Neurosurgical Patient 77
   Gwen J. Stephens
   Mickey C. Parsons

Hypophysectomy for Diabetic Retinopathy 89
   Sharon M. Stowe

Cerebellar Stimulation: Pacing the Brain 101
   Bridget C. Loetterle
   Maisie Rogers
   Tina Valdner
   Carmen Mason
   Ina Christian
   Wayne Andreesen

Myasthenia Gravis 107
   Joan Stackhouse

Caring for a Young Addict with Tetanus 116
   Catherine M. Boyer

Amyotrophic Lateral Sclerosis 121
   Mary A. Boyle
   Rudy L. Ciuca

SECTION IV: Traumatic Neurological Damage: Acute Care and Rehabilitation

Craniocerebral Trauma 131
   Ann Hinkhouse

Respiratory Changes in Head Injury 139
   L. Claire Parsons

Nursing Rehabilitation After Severe Head Trauma 149
   Edith Norsworthy

A Paraplegic Reflects 159
   Ray Burridge

Automonic Hyperreflexia 163
   Delycia Feustel

Sexual Function in Traumatic Paraplegia and Quadriplegia 169
    A. Estin Comarr
    Bernice B. Gunderson

Sexuality and the Severely Disabled Person 182
    Jim Smith
    Bonnie Bullough

Janie Remembered 191
    Mattie Tolley

SECTION V: **Cerebral Vascular Disease: Acute Care and Rehabilitation**

Transient Ischemic Attacks 195
    Margaret R. Keller
    B. Lionel Truscott

Stroke 200
    Ann M. Jacobansky

Subarachnoid Hemorrhage 208
    Marjorie Maddox

Motor Skill Rehabilitation for Hemiplegic Patients 215
    Marjorie Pfaudler

Soft or Hard Devices to Position Hands? 225
    Nancy Dayhoff

Feeding Techniques for Dysphagic Patients 232
    Terry Weiler Gaffney
    Rosemary Peterson Campbell

Working with Dysphasic Patients 237
    Linda Hagen Belt

Aphasic Patients Talk Back 243
    Madge Skelly

Resocializing . . . Through a Stroke Club 248
    Helen M. Falknor
    Beverly J. Harris

Autumn Months, Autumn Years 253
    Marion B. Dolan

Section I
Assessment and Diagnostic Testing

A person's ability to function physically or mentally may be altered by neurological disorders. Identification of such difficulties enables the nurse to plan care which promotes the safety and well-being of her patient and which may contribute to his rehabilitation. The first three articles in this section provide some guidelines for assessing patients' physical and mental capacities.

The remaining articles concern the preparation of patients for various diagnostic procedures. These authors stress the necessity for adequate pre-procedure teaching to alleviate the patient's anxiety and avoid the need for repeat examinations.

Assessing Station and Gait

MARIAH SNYDER • REBECCA BAUM

> *These authors developed a tool to evaluate neurological patients' station and gait. After determining that the tool was both valid and reliable, they tested it. Ten pairs of nurses were assigned at random to evaluate patients. One nurse in each pair used the tool; the other did not. Questionnaires answered by the nurses indicated that the tool made a statistically significant difference in nurses' ability to assess disturbances in station and gait.*

Many neurological disorders cause various disturbances in station and gait. A person with hemiplegia may shuffle on the affected side. A patient with cerebellar disease may compensate by adopting a wide, waddling gait. At times, nurses' expectations for the hospitalized patient who has a station or gait disturbance may exceed his abilities. On other occasions, he is given complete assistance when he is quite able to move independently. Establishing the baseline abilities of a newly hospitalized neurological patient should be an integral part of his care.

We developed and tested a tool which helps nurses assess the patient's level of ability and disability so that nursing intervention can be appropriate.

In addition to general questions about his gait, the assessment includes observation of the patient in a variety of situations. Any paralysis, paresis, or atrophy can be detected by observing the patient as he lies in bed. This information is helpful in determining possible problems in

---

MS. SNYDER (B.S.N., College of St. Teresa, Winona, Minn.; MSN., University of Pennsylvania, Philadelphia) is an instructor in the school of nursing, University of Wisconsin, Eau Claire. MS. BAUM (B.S.N., M.S.N., University of Pennsylvania, Philadelphia) works part time at Norfolk General Hospital, Va.

Patient's Name _____
Date _____
Nurse _____

General information

1. How long has the patient had difficulty in walking?
2. Is the difficulty increasing? — Yes / No
3. Is it worse at a particular time of day? — Yes / No
   If yes, when? _____
4. How far can he walk (around one block, several blocks, only in the house)? _____
5. Is it painful to walk? — Yes / No
   If yes, where is the pain? _____
6. Does he use an aid (cane, walker, crutch)? — Yes / No
   If yes, when does he use it? _____

Observe the patient lying in bed.

7. Is he able to move his legs in bed? — Yes / No
   If no, which leg is he unable to move? — Right / Left
8. Do his legs appear to be equal in size? — Yes / No
   If no, describe the inequality. _____

Ask the patient to sit with his legs over the side of the bed.

9. Does the patient need assistance in sitting up? — Yes / No
   If yes, describe. _____

Ask the patient to stand in one spot for a minute.

10. Does he require assistance to stand? — Yes / No
    If yes, describe. _____
11. Is he able to stand for one minute? — Yes / No
12. Does he stand erect (are his hips directly over his legs)? — Yes / No
13. Does he reach for support? — Yes / No
14. Does he sway while standing? — Yes / No
    If yes, in what direction? — Right / Left
    — Front / Back

Ask the patient to close his eyes.

15. Does he sway with his eyes closed? — Yes / No
    If yes, in what direction? — Right / Left
    — Front / Back

Ask the patient to walk to a chair placed 10 feet away.

16. Is he able to walk without assistance? — Yes / No
    If no, describe. _____
17. Does he walk erect? — Yes / No
    If no, in what direction does he lean? — Right / Left
    — Front / Back

CONTEMPORARY NURSING SERIES

18.	Does he walk with his feet apart (wide-based gait)?	Yes	No
19.	Does he cross his feet (scissors gait) when he walks?	Yes	No
20.	Does he shuffle his feet when he walks?	Yes	No
21.	Does he walk with a limp?	Yes	No
	If yes, which leg does he favor?	Right	Left
22.	Does he drag his foot when he walks?	Yes	No
	If yes, which foot?	Right	Left
23.	Does he slap his feet down?	Yes	No
	If yes, which foot?	Right	Left
24.	Does he swing his arms freely?	Yes	No

Ask the patient to walk clockwise and then counter-clockwise around the chair.

25.	Can he turn clockwise without support?	Yes	No
	If no, describe. ————————		
26.	Can he turn counterclockwise without support?	Yes	No
	If no, describe. ————————		

Thank the patient for his cooperation. Observe him as he walks to his bed. If he uses an aid, give it to him. Continue to observe him without asking questions.

27.	Does he keep his eyes on the floor while he walks?	Yes	No
28.	Does his gait change in any manner from what you previously observed?	Yes	No
	If yes, describe. ————————		
29.	Does he have difficulty starting to walk?	Yes	No
30.	Does he walk at an even pace?	Yes	No
	If no, describe. ————————		

From your observations, determine the patient's need for assistance.

31.	The patient is able to stand without assistance for daily weights or to void.	Yes	No
32.	He can walk to the bathroom without assistance and use the facilities.	Yes	No
33.	He needs assistance at all times when walking.	Yes	No
34.	He requires assistance on a particular side.	Yes	No
		Right	Left
35.	He needs reminders for safety (reminder to walk slowly).	Yes	No
36.	He can walk to the bathroom using environmental supports (chairs, wall), or an aid such as a walker or a cane.	Yes	No
	He uses these aids (list):		

mobilization. The patient's ability to sit up unassisted gives clues to his ability to feed himself. His stability when standing helps the nurse decide how much independence he can safely assume. For example, if the patient sways to one side, he will need assistance on that side when he walks.

His walking patterns indicate the need for a special environmental arrangement in the hospital and serve as a basis for future teaching about the home environment. For example, obstacles such as mats are unsafe for the patient who shuffles. Also, the patient's ability to turn helps to determine how independently he can use the bathroom without assistance.

Evaluation tools are beneficial only if their use leads to better planning and delivery of care. Conclusions drawn from an assessment of gait and stance can be used to evaluate exacerbations or remissions in patients with certain neurological disorders and should be the basis of planned interventions to ensure the patient's safety and independence.

Guidelines for the Care of Confused Patients

MAGDALENA MORRIS • MARTHA RHODES

A nurse who can differentiate between organic and functional confusion is in a position to prevent some patients from becoming even more confused and others from being subject to unnecessary medication or restraints.

The second night after Mr. M.'s surgery, he became confused, agitated, and said he was seeing bugs crawl over his bedspread. Periodically, screams were heard from his room. The night nurse said, when she was asked what was wrong with Mr. M., "He's gone crazy," and added that she had to restrain him. "There was nothing else we could do."

Ms. P., a 48-year-old woman who had become depressed following a period of severe emotional stress, was diagnosed as having an involutional psychosis. When she failed to respond to conventional psychiatric treatment after several weeks on the ward, the nursing staff began to say, "There is nothing else we can do."

It is not true that there is "nothing else we can do." One of the first things a nurse can do is determine whether a patient is functionally or organically confused.

MS. MORRIS *(Presbyterian-University Hospital School of Nursing, Pittsburgh) has had experience in medical, neurosurgical, and psychiatric nursing. She is now a student in the baccalaureate program at the University of California School of Nursing in San Francisco. For two and one-half years, she was a staff nurse on the unit where Ms. Rhodes was supervising nurse.* MS. RHODES *(Scott and White Memorial Hospital School of Nursing, Temple, Tex.) has had extensive clinical experience as a nurse in a large state psychiatric hospital, a psychiatric admission unit at a county hospital, and as a supervising nurse on an acute psychiatric admission unit. She is now teaching psychiatric technicians at Napa College, Calif.*

Confusion is defined as a state of disorder and mental derangement. Attention span, memory, retention and recall, and sensory perceptions are affected.(1).

Organic confusion is a mental disorder which is due to such physical causes as electrolyte imbalance, infection, alcohol withdrawal (a toxic factor), cerebral disease, and respiratory disturbances(2).

Functional confusion is a mental disorder (such as schizophrenia) which is due to psychosocial, psychosexual, and developmental factors.

GUIDELINES FOR DIFFERENTIATING ORGANIC FROM FUNCTIONAL CONFUSION

FACTOR	ORGANIC CONFUSION	FUNCTIONAL CONFUSION
Memory Impairment	Recent more impaired than remote	No consistent difference between recent and remote
Disorientation:		
Time	Within own lifetime or reasonably near future	May not be related to patient's lifetime
Place	Familiar place or one where patient might easily be	Bizarre or unfamiliar places
Person	Sense of identity usually preserved	Sense of identity diminished
	Misidentification of others as familiar	Misidentification of others based on delusional system
Hallucinations	Visual, vivid. Animals and insects common	Auditory more frequent Bizarre and symbolic
Illusions	Common	Not prominent
Delusions	Concerns everyday occurrences and people	Bizarre and symbolic
Confused	Spotty confusion. Clear intervals mixed with confused episodes	More consistent
	Worse at night	No tendency to become worse at night

At this point you may be asking why it is important for nurses to assess the type of confusion. Primarily, it is because nurses are with patients a greater amount of time than physicians and, therefore, can be instrumental in changing therapy early. If a nurse notices a patient exhibiting early signs of organic confusion, she can withhold such medications as barbiturates, which tend to increase confusion, or withhold tap water enemas for elderly patients, whose confusion may be due to electrolyte imbalance, and then report her observations to the physician(3). Withholding medications and treatment may prevent progression of the confusion until the physician has a chance to evaluate the patient. And, if confusion is noticed in its early stages restraints may be unnecessary.

If a nurse can recognize that a patient's confusion may be due to organic causes, she is able to make wiser judgments about when to give Thorazine instead of barbiturates at bedtime.

The ability to differentiate between organic confusion and functional confusion permits nurses to tailor their intervention to specific patient problems.

Nursing care approaches toward the organically confused patient and the functionally confused patient do differ. For example, with the patient who is organically confused, a nurse must be prepared to answer questions repeatedly in short, simple sentences. She should demonstrate nonverbally and concretely what she is trying to convey to him. She should tell him when she does not understand what he is talking about. She should not support his disorientation, but should try to help him as frequently as necessary to become oriented through the use of clocks, calendars, signs, and written and verbal reminders.

Generally, with functionally confused patients, the nursing approach will vary with the patient's behavior and the psychodynamics of his illness. Frequently, trying to help schizophrenic patients become oriented in a direct way may oppose their delusional system; relating to their healthier level may prove more beneficial. Answering certain ritualized questions over and over again tends to perpetuate unhealthy behavior patterns. For this reason, it may be better to tell a patient that you do not wish to discuss delusional material with him.

Subtle qualities of symptoms are important for differentiating between organic and functional confusion. Patients whom nurses frequently label "confused" or "crazy" or "unmanageable" often exhibit poor memory, disorientation, delusions, hallucinations, and other psychotic symptoms. Although the symptoms of a patient who is organically confused may superficially appear to be as bizarre as those of a functionally confused patient, closer inspection of the quality of the symptom may reveal important differences.

One approach is to view the patient's behavior as an attempt to interpret, explain, and manage his environment. The functionally confused patient tends to interpret events in the light of his private inner experiences and to express his interpretations in a symbolic and bizarre fashion.

The organically confused patient tends to interpret and explain events in the light of his own previous everyday experiences and to couch his explanations in conventional language.

Impairment of memory is a major symptom which helps to separate organic disorders from all others(4). It is responsible for a large part of a patient's failure to follow directions and cooperate in his care. Characteristically, an organically confused patient exhibits impaired recent memory, combined with preservation of remote memory. He may be unable to relate the details of events that have occurred only a few minutes before, yet recall in considerable detail events which took place far in the past. Memory loss seems to arise from disorganization of cerebral function; amnesia does not occur as a mechanism to protect him from painful memories.

Memory loss in a patient with a functional disorder, however, seems to be a protective mechanism. Recent or remote memory may be impaired, depending upon when the painful experience occurred.

Disorientation is another prominent feature of organic confusion. It is less commonly exhibited by patients suffering from functional disorders, but it can occur. When asked to give the date and hour, the organically confused patient may give a variety of answers. He may be only a few hours off the mark, or he may give a date several years in the past. He nearly always gives a date within his own lifetime or the very near future. But the patient with a functional disorder who is confused about time will frequently give a date many years before he was born or one in a future century.

The organically confused patient usually has some disorientation regarding place. Frequently, he thinks he is at home, in a city other than the one where he actually is, or in a motel. If he is in a large psychiatric ward, he frequently thinks he is in prison, but, wherever he may think he is, it is a place where he actually has been or easily could be. Such a patient also often loses his way if he leaves his room. The patient with a functional disorder who is disoriented about place, on the other hand, will probably name a place that has a symbolic meaning for him. He may say he is in hell, on the moon, or on a nonexistent planet.

The organically confused patient usually knows his own name and knows that he is one person with one continuing life history, even if he cannot remember details. Patients with functional disorders sometimes say that they feel like two persons, or that they are someone other than their real selves.

People and their relationship to him are a problem for an organically confused patient. He will frequently misidentify persons as those familiar to him. For example, he may insist that the male nurse is his nephew and the female nurse is the cashier at the local supermarket. The patient with a functional disorder, by contrast, will tend to misidentify others as enemies or someone who fits in with his delusional system, and he is not likely to say that he has seen them before.

If an organically confused patient is hallucinating, he most probably will have visual hallucinations. He usually will see something he has seen before or could conceivably have seen; frequently, he sees animals or insects. On closer inspection, such a patient is often found to be experiencing illusions, misinterpreting actual external stimuli, rather than having hallucinations. For example, a bit of lint becomes an insect marching across his bed; the cord to his bathrobe becomes a snake. The patient with a functional disorder will, instead, describe auditory hallucinations. Visual hallucinations are rare, and when they do occur, they lack the vividness and concreteness of those experienced by the organically ill patient(5).

The delusions of an organically confused patient are seldom as elaborate or as symbolic as those of the patient with a functional disorder. It is unlikely that an organically confused patient will state that he has to leave the hospital immediately in order to save the world. It is more likely for him to say that he has to go home to mow the lawn or to get ready to go to work. He is unlikely to say that Napoleon is waiting to consult him, but he is apt to say that his brother is just outside the door, ready to take him home.

If there is a common thread through all the organically confused individual's behavior, it seems to be a consistent attempt to use the familiar and the commonplace to make some sense out of what is going on. He searches his environment for cues to help him interpret what is happening to him. He may try to memorize the number of his room, and he will often be seen anxiously looking for signs on doors or for clocks and calendars. His behavior and affect are usually consistent with his evaluation of the situation. If he thinks he is at work, he will go through the motions that his job requires and become upset when anyone tries to interfere. If he thinks he is at home and realizes that the nurse is a stranger, he may become indignant and even abusive. If he thinks he is in jail, he may think that the nurse is a relative and beg her to remove him from that terrible place. There is no such consistency for the functionally confused patient. His behavior and affect bear little relation to his stated beliefs.

No organically confused patient will exhibit all the behaviors described and no patient will exhibit such behavior all of the time. A common characteristic of the organically confused patient is that his confusion occurs at intervals. As a result, he is quite clear and cooperative one moment and totally confused the next. It is at night, when there are fewer external cues to guide him, that the intensity of his confusion increases.

Now, let us return to Mr. M. and Ms. P. Mr. M. was a 72-year-old man who had had surgery for repair of a broken hip. He had had a temperature of 100.4 F. through the second postoperative day. That second morning, he did not remember things five minutes after the nurses had explained them to him. After his wife visited him, Mr. M. thought he was at home and referred to the evening nurse as his niece. The evening nurse gave him Seconal at bedtime, but he became agitated rather than drowsy. Later that night, his behavior changed to severe agitation and profound confusion. He thought the spots on his bedspread were bugs; he became very frightened.

During evening visiting hours, his wife mentioned that for a few days before admission, Mr. M. had had little to eat or drink. On the morning after his confusion, he was very dehydrated and had low serum potassium levels. Almost immediately after intravenous fluid replacement with potassium chloride, his confusion subsided. Had the nurses identified his confusion as organic in its early stages, fluid replacement may have been initiated sooner. If the evening nurse had given him Thorazine instead of Seconal, perhaps he might have been spared some of his agitation and fear through the night.

A review of Ms. P.'s behavior revealed that she still could not find the way from her own room to the dining room, that she appeared unable to remember the few sequential steps of a simple occupational therapy project, and that she often did not know the exact date. Even after several days in the unit, she did not know the names of the nursing staff and often called them by the names of her children. Ms. P. was diagnosed as having an involutional psychosis. When she did not respond to treatment, her physician did extensive tests which indicated that she was suffering from the early stages of a cerebral degenerative disease. In this instance, had the nursing staff noted her memory lapses for recent events and her disorientation of time and place and if they had known that the quality of her symptoms were suggestive of organic confusion, the diagnostic workup might have occurred sooner and some preventive measures initiated.

In conclusion, we believe our guidelines are valuable in differentiating between organic and functional confusion, and that such differentiation is an important aspect of nursing assessment and care. Our guidelines are only a rough tool, however, which need to be tried out in a controlled situation.

REFERENCES

1. WEYMOUTH, L. T. Nursing care of the so-called confused patient. *Nurs.Clin.NorthAm.* 3:709-715. Dec. 1968.
2. KAUFER, C. Etiology of consciousness disturbances in surgery. *Minn.Med.* 51:1509-1515, Nov. 1968.
3. NOYES, A. P., AND KOLB, L. C. *Modern Clinical Psychiatry.* 7th ed. Philadelphia. W. B. Saunders Co., 1968.
4. NATHAN, P. E., AND OTHERS. Systems analytic model of diagnosis; Part 6. Improved diagnostic validity from median data. *J.Clin. Psychol.* 25:370-375. Apr. 1969.
5. ―――. Systems analytic model of diagnosis; Part 2. Diagnostic valdity of abnormal perceptual behavior. *J.Clin.Psychol.* 25: 115-119, Feb. 1969.

BIBLIOGRAPHY

GERDES, LENORE. Confused or delirious patient. *Am.J.Nurs.* 68:1228-1233. June 1968.

MCCOWN, P. P., AND WURM, ELIZABETH. Orienting the disoriented. *Am.J.Nurs.* 65-118-119, Apr. 1965.

NATHAN, P. E. Systems analytic model of diagnosis; Part 5. Diagnostic validity of disordered consciousness. *J.Clin.Psychol.* 25:243-246, Mar. 1969.

PATRICK, M. L. Care of the confused elderly patient. *Am.J.Nurs.* 67:2536-2539. Dec. 1967.

TYLER, C. R. Nurse's influence on Mr. Brown's orientation. IN *ANA (Regional) Clinical Conferences, 1969.* New York. Appelton-Century-Crofts, 1970, pp. 150-156.

Optokinetic Nystagmus

GEORGE L. LARSEN

> *The patient who can describe the steps involved in a motor task, but cannot perform the task, may have constructional apraxia. A simple test can confirm this diagnosis and provide information regarding the patient's prognosis.*

The stroke patient has perplexing problems. Often he appears bright and alert, seems to understand what you say to him, and can even tell you what he is expected to do but then cannot proceed. Often this patient has right hemispheric brain damage and a left-sided paralysis. If a tray is placed in front of him, he may not be able to eat because he can't get himself organized to take the steps involved in eating. If given his clothes, he may not be able to dress even though he can tell you what is entailed. In the Speech Pathology Unit at the Veterans Administration Hospital in Seattle, we call this problem constructional apraxia, a disorder of motor-perceptual planning for solving problems.

Optokinetic nystagmus testing is a physiologic tool which may be used in evaluating patients who suffer constructional apraxia, and the visual neglect and denial phenomenon that usually accompany it. Visual neglect is on the mild end of a pathologic continuum representing the person's cortical appreciation that he and his environment exist. Denial is on the severe end of the continuum. These terms are not to be confused with descriptions of emotional states, but are, rather, behavioral deficits asso-

---

DR. LARSEN *(Ph.D., University of Washington, Seattle) is chief of speech pathology at Seattle VA Hospital. He is also a clinical associate in the College of Arts and Sciences' program in audiology and speech pathology, the School of Medicine's department of rehabilitation medicine, and the School of Nursing at the University of Washington.*

ciated with cortical pathology. They are particularly useful in predicting a patient's ability to learn and retain new information that requires a motor plan.

Optokinetic nystagmus is a physiologic response that may be elicited both horizontally and vertically. When the eyes are fixed on a moving object, such as rotating drum or the landscape as observed from a moving vehicle, they slowly follow the object and then rapidly return to the side from which the movement came. Reduction or loss of this response on one side may result from a lesion of the contralateral temporal or parietal cortex, and this has been used as a diagnostic test(1).

There are two commonly employed means of testing the optokinetic responses. The classic method is by means of an optokinetic drum. This is usually a 12-inch drum with alternating black and white stripes, although a series of other targets may be used if desired. The drum is held about 20 inches from the patient and rotated to produce a movement of about six to eight frames per second. A second technique is use of an optokinetic tape. One can easily construct such a tape by drawing heavy black lines, about ½ inch apart and about ½ inch wide on a length of 1-inch wide cloth tape. Another simple tape to use is a cloth measuring tape with large black numerals printed on it. Several such tapes of different sizes and patterns can be kept available. Material with any bright pattern may be cut into tapes 40 inches long.

Targets are presented to the patient by moving the tape slowly in front of him, from his left to his right, then from his right to his left, from below upward and from above downward. This tests for optokinetic responses in both the vertical and horizontal positions. The response observed is graded from 0 to 4+ in the direction from which the movement originated, with 4+ being a brisk, normal response, and 1+ being the least discernible response. Thus R 4+, L 4+, U 4+, D 4+ is the response recorded(2). Diminished or lost optokinetic responses from one side usually imply a lesion in the temporal or parietal cortex in the contralateral side, since the visual associational cortex controls normal fixation and release responses.

Our experience indicates that subjects with left hemiplegia who have impaired optokinetic responses from the left often suffer constructional apraxia. For them, the speech pathologist must structure language units in a way that expedites rehabilitation by using speech as a support system for the impaired motor system. However, if a patient continues to have absent optokinetic responses throughout his rehabilitation program, he frequently is unable to initiate new motor tasks or to retain newly taught motor tasks. Patients suffering aphasia and right hemiplegia may also have impaired optokinetic responses from the right side. This is less common, however, since the language cortex apparently provides a secondary operational system for this physiologic response. The possible relationship between the severity of aphasia and reduced optokinetic responses has yet to be explored.

Optokinetic nystagmus testing also permits differentiation of the neglect-denial phenomenon from homonymous hemianopia. Homonymous hemianopia is the loss of vision in half the field of each eye. With this condition, nystagmus jerks will appear as soon as the targets are presented in the preserved half of the visual field. The qualitive score will be equal to the nystagmus jerks elicited from the non-involved side. Optokinetic nystagmus testing is not a substitute for neurological diagnosis or prognosis but an additional tool that nurses can use to predict prognosis and plan care.

REFERENCES
1. WATSON, J. N. Essentials of Neurology. 3d ed. Philadelphia, J. B. Lippincott Co., 1971.
2. SMITH, J. L. *Optokinetic Nystagmus.* Springfield, Ill. Charles C Thomas, Publisher, 1963.

P.E.G. and Angiography: A Patient's Sensations

CAROL ANN BLACKWELL

Not knowing what to expect during an invasive diagnostic procedure can add to the fears patients already have about what the test may reveal.

In December of 1972, without warning, I had a grand mal seizure. I had been driving our family car for two hours. Ten minutes after my husband took the wheel, I began to feel very distant from everything around me. Forty-five minutes later, I was in an ambulance. All I could think was, "I'm a nurse, not a patient."

I was finishing the first semester in a graduate nursing program. This could not be happening to me. But I *was* a patient, and the brain scan done at the infirmary was abnormal.

Since then, I have had three craniotomies for a brain tumor, courses of chemotherapy and radiation therapy, and rehabilitative speech and occupational therapy. Because I found the carotid arteriogram and the pneumoencephalogram very traumatic, I believe that medical personnel need to know more about patients' sensations during these tests so that they prepare patients for the events and physical sensations that they entail. Prior knowledge of the sensory aspects of both procedures would have greatly reduced my anxiety and fears.

An arteriogram is a contrast x-ray in which a radiopaque substance is injected into a major artery to permit visualization of a specific blood

---

MS. BLACKWELL (B.S.N., University of North Carolina at Chapel Hill, Chapel Hill) is a graduate student at the University of North Carolina at Chapel Hill. She has worked in a pediatric intensive care unit at Texas Children's Hospital, Houston. Her fourth craniotomy, for excision of scar tissue, showed no visible signs of tumor recurrence. She thanks Maureen Callahan, R.N. for her help in preparing the neurophysiological aspects of this article.

vessel system. The serial films, taken after dye is injected into the carotid artery, show filling of the cerebral vessels and are useful in the differential diagnosis of tumors, hematomas, arteriovenous, malformations, and aneurysms.

My knowledge of carotid arteriography was limited, and my fear was great. I had heard about a patient who died after an anaphylactic reaction to the dye. As I signed the permit, I was informed of the possibility of having a stroke. Death and stroke weighed heavily on my mind as I was medicated and taken almost immediately to the neuroradiology department.

Everything was happening too fast. As I lay waiting on the stretcher in the busy hallway, two technicians explained how I would feel when the dye was injected. In the room I could see people setting up trays and equipment. Within minutes, I was there: flat on my back on a cold table, my forehead taped down to the table, my hands restrained, my neck hyperextended. I saw the tracheostomy and arrest trays on my right, and I dreaded each radiologist who palpated my neck as he passed.

Insertion of the needle into my left carotid artery was extremely frightening. The Xylocaine was injected millimeter by millimeter until I felt sure that the needle had pierced the back of my neck. Then, when the area was numb, the doctor inserted a one-and-three-quarter-inch, 18-gauge stylet, which caused a large spurt of arterial blood. It hurt for only a few seconds, but I was extremely anxious because the needle felt so close to my trachea. I knew I should not breathe deeply because the neuroradiologist had emphasized that talking, coughing, or movement might dislodge the catheter.

I felt most alone after the protective shield was lowered and suspended over my entire body. Only my head was my own. All the technicians had left the room and the doctor told me he was ready for the first injection. "Shoot!" shouted the neuroradiologist. The bolus of dye rushed into my brain and I heard the fast clackey-clack of the machine. The combination was terrifying. I began to feel burning directly behind my left eye and, even though my eyes were closed, I saw bright orange branches on the surface of my eyelids. Just when the burning seemed overwhelming, it subsided. The whole injection process probably took four to six seconds. I was still alive—no anaphylaxis, no stroke.

After the first injection, I became aware of my arterial pulsations, visible in the plastic tubing. The doctor was irrigating the tube constantly, to prevent clot formation. The saline felt cool around my left chin, lips, and cheek. It caused no discomfort.

The third injection of dye was the last, and removal of the catheter caused another large spurt of arterial blood. The doctor quickly applied a pressure dressing which he held firmly in place for a long 10 minutes. It hurt. My whole neck felt as though it was in spasm. Not only was this painful, it was also alarming because I could not breathe well, a feeling that persisted all night.

Back in my room, the nurse applied an ice pack to my neck, checked my vital signs every 15 minutes, and asked if I was having any difficulty swallowing or breathing. I was to lie flat for eight hours but could have clear liquids. The arteriogram was over, but I was very much aware of the trachesostomy tray and suction setup at my bedside. I could not imagine a more traumatic experience, but there were more difficult times to come.

A pneumoencephalogram is a neurodiagnostic, contrast study in which a lumbar puncture is done, cerebrospinal fluid removed, and air injected into the subarachnoid space. This air fills the cerebral ventricular system and appears as shadows on x-ray film. Dilations, distortions in shape, and filling defects in the ventricles are visualized and interpeted for the differential diagnosis of tumor, hematomas, hydrocephalus, and other abnormalities involving the cerebrospinal fluid pathways.

I had a pneumoencephalogram the day after the carotid arteriogram. I was surprised to have to give permission for both the P.E.G. and a craniotomy. The craniotomy was presented as a very matter-of-fact possibility. There was a remote chance that the air injection would change the pressure within my head. If I was not able to accommodate to this change, an emergency craniotomy would be necessary to relieve the increased pressure. After signing the permission, I had all night to become anxious and think of questions about the test. The nurse who gave me my preprocedure medications said that patients found this an extremely painful test and that they had had headaches for several days afterward. I had never in my life hurt for a long time—what would this be like?

The pneumonencephalogram room was similar to the room used for my carotid arteriogram. I was less anxious because the same doctors and technicians were there. Yet I could not forget what the nurse had told me, though I managed to persuade myself that nothing could be that bad. I was positioned sitting upright in a straight-backed chair, my forehead resting on a hard x-ray plate, both arms strapped at my sides. I felt boxed in, trapped.

The neuroradiologist told me there would be a stinging sensation when he injected the Xylocaine in the small of my back. As the local took effect, he explained that he would do a lumbar puncture and inject air into my spinal column and ventricles. He would talk to me constantly, he said, because patients frequently faint during the procedure. I could expect to perspire and be nauseated. With this information I suddenly began to perspire. I was frightened again.

With the injection of the first 10 cc. of air I could feel bubbles traveling up my spine. Pain radiated from my spinal column and around my rib cage. When the air reached the ventricles, I experienced a throbbing much like a sinus headache. The pain increased when the doctor moved my head from side to side. I heard a sloshing noise in the middle of my brain, a sound that would continue for 48 hours, until all the air was absorbed.

X-rays were taken with my head in various positions. Then I had to wait while the doctors looked at the films on the view boxes. I could hear them talking, but too softly for me to catch the words. The waiting was very difficult because my head was really beginning to hurt.

The next 10 cc. injection was excruciating. The positions my head was put in seemed unbearable. Once again I felt the tiny air bubbles traveling up my spine and heard the now deafening, sloshing sounds. The wait for the films to be developed seemed endless. I was perspiring, hot one minute and cold the next. "How much more?" I asked. A technician removed my restraints and gave me a moist gauze pad to suck on—a beautiful pause in the midst of pain.

During the injection of the last 10 cc., I was praying that I would faint, but I couldn't think how and I was too exhausted to try.

One year, five operations, and 34 radiation treatments later, the P.E.G. still stands out as causing the most intense pain I have ever felt. I did not even notice the removal of the lumbar puncture needle. More films were taken, and then I was lifted onto a stretcher so I could be positioned in still another way. My head hung off the end of the stretcher, and I felt powerless to move it. A technician supported my head as I waited for the films to be developed.

At last I was lifted to the stretcher that would take me to my room. Instead, I was left in the hallway. I vaguely remember someone asking, "Do you hurt enough to need codeine?" What a ridiculous question! But not so absurd as his statement, "Well, I'm not really sure where to give this." I was frightened and angered to be in the hands of a doctor who did not know where to give a shot.

Once back in my room, my family and friends helped me to move my head and to be as comfortable as possible. The quiet and darkness were peaceful. I was relieved to be through the test at last. I had survived. The diagnosis was clear. I would have surgery in the morning.

My experiences as a patient and nurse have convinced me that every

INFORMATION FOR PATIENTS

Carotid Arteriogram

Before the procedure, the patient can expect
To sign a permit, take nothing by mouth after midnight, and receive preprocedure medications.

Information about the test
Appearance of x-ray room and machinery.
Flat position on hard table.
Head and hands restrained by tape.
Needle inserted after local anesthetic takes effect.
Spurt of arterial blood after needle insertion.
Needle feels close to trachea; may cause some difficulty breathing.
Shield is lowered, covering body from neck down; feeling of body loss.
Dye feels warm at first, becomes hotter; burning sensation lasts about 4-6 seconds.
Noises during test; radiologist calls "Shoot," clackety-clack sound of plate changer.

After the procedure, the patient can expect
To remain flat in bed for eight hours, but turn from side to side.
Soreness at injection site, with swelling, possible hematoma, and effect on breathing and swallowing.
Frequent vital sign checks, emergency equipment kept near by as a precaution.
Frequent neurological checks, especially of movement and strength of extremities.

Pneumoencephalogram

Before the procedure, the patient can expect
To sign a permit for both the PEG and a craniotomy, take nothing by mouth after midnight, and receive preprocedure medications.

Information about the test
Appearance of x-ray room and machinery.
Upright position in straight-backed chair.
Arms restrained at sides.
X-ray plate in front of face; feeling of being trapped.
LP performed after local anesthetic takes effect.
Air is injected and can be felt rising up spine to ventricles.
Head constantly repositioned; sloshing sound of air in ventricles.
Several waits for processing of x-rays.
Difficult to move head; feels heavy.

After the procedure, the patient can expect
To remain flat in bed for 12 to 24 hours, but turn from side to side, and hear air moving in ventricles.
Possible headache, photophobia, nausea and vomiting, chills, low-grade fever.
Analgesics, antiemetics, fluids, and dark environment to relieve discomfort.
Frequent checking of vital signs.
Frequent neurological checks, especially of level of consciousness.

patient should be given the opportunity to become familiar with the sensations he may have during a carotid arteriogram or a pneumoencephalogram. After evaluating the patient's need to know and ability to understand, the nurse should share information about these tests with the patient far enough in advance to answer whatever questions he may have.

Preparing a Patient for EEG

DONALD SHEARER • BETTY COLLINS • DONNELL CREEL

Preprocedure teaching is also important for persons undergoing even relatively simple, noninvasive tests.

Most diagnostic examinations are completed more successfully if the patient is prepared for them. Shoddy preparatory techniques often leave the patient apprehensive, nervous, and uncooperative, and cause expensive and time-consuming repeat examinations. Patients who are scheduled for electroencephalographic examinations must be properly prepared so that they are comfortable, relaxed, and able to cooperate throughout the procedure.

The patient's physician should begin the preparation when he tells the patient that he is to have an EEG. At this time the physician should briefly explain an EEG's purpose, what results can be expected from it, and that it is a useful and painless procedure. This can do much to eliminate unnecessary fear and apprehension. Without a patient's relaxed cooperation, an artifact-free EEG cannot be obtained.

Physical preparation is very important. All anticonvulsants, tranquilizers, and stimulants, including alcohol, should be discontinued for at least 24 to 48 hours before the EEG. These medications can alter the basic wave patterns of the EEG markedly, and may mask or suppress the abnormal brain waves and discharges of seizure disorders, behavior problems, and brain lesions.

The patient may eat his normal meals before the EEG, except for coffee, tea, and cola drinks. These tend to have a slight stimulatory

---

MR. SHEARER *is a research EEG technician in neuropsychology research at Veterans Administration Hospital, Salt Lake City, Utah.* MS. COLLINS *is chief EEG technician at Veterans Administration Hospital, Phoenix, Ariz.* DR. CREEL *(Ph.D, University of Utah, Salt Lake City) is director of the neuropsychological research laboratories at Veterans Administration Hospital, Phoenix, Ariz.*

effect. No meals should be skipped, as this can alter blood sugar levels, and hypoglycemia can change normal brain wave patterns.

The patient should go to bed relatively late the night before the test and rise early in the morning. Napping before the EEG is rigidly prohibited, even for infants and young children. This is done to ensure that the patient will come to the EEG laboratory so tired that he can fall asleep without medication during the recording of the EEG. Also, sleep deprivation may help evoke abnormal brain potentials.

When the EEG is ordered, however, the physician should prescribe a light, short-acting sleeping medication (such as chloral hydrate) to be used, if necessary, before the recording of drowsing and sleep patterns. Because these drugs alter the brain wave patterns they should be given only as a last resort. Recording a drowsy and sleep EEG is important, however, because some abnormal brain waves and discharges are emitted only when the patient is drowsing or asleep.

The patient's hair should be washed well with a mild soap shampoo the night before or several hours before the EEG. The hair should be completely dry at the time of the test and oils, spray, or lotions should not be applied until after it is completed.

The psychological preparation is often more important than the physical. Apprehension, nervousness, and fear can alter and contaminate the recording.

There is rarely, if ever, a good reason not to explain the procedure completely to the patient. A person who knows where he is going and what is to happen is more apt to cooperate than is the patient who is suddenly told to get ready for an EEG.

The EEG can be compared to a radio or TV station, with the patient as the station and the EEG instrument as the radio or TV receiving set. This explanation often works well with young children. The EEG can also be compared to an electrocardiogram if the patient has had this examination. Essentially, the EEG is a recording ot the brain's electrical output. The patient should know that it is not a test of intelligence or sanity, will not hypnotize him, and cannot read his mind. A final point is that the equipment will not shock him. All the electricity involved in the examination is provided by the patient's own brain in miniscule amounts that are measured in millionths of a volt.

Fears of physical pain should be eliminated by a thorough explanation of the testing procedure. This is usually done by the technician, but the nursing staff can pave the way by briefly explaining the procedure. Ordinarily, surface scalp electrodes are used. However, some EEG laboratories use subdermal needle electrodes, so find out what type are employed in your hospital laboratory. A patient who was told he would have surface scalp electrodes and then receives the subdermal needle type can be a little irritable with the technician.

If surface electrodes are used, the technician cleans the scalp under the electrodes with alcohol or acetone to remove any dead skin or oil and then attaches 19 to 21 electrodes to the scalp with a paste-like substance that helps conduct the brain waves from the area beneath the electrodes. The electrode is then covered by a glue-like material to ensure that it does not shift its position on the scalp. A shampoo will remove the conductive paste and glue after the test. Subdermal needle electrodes are inserted into the scalp. This is done with a minimum of discomfort, but many patients fear needles, no matter how small. Therefore, these electrodes are not as popular as surface electrodes.

Patient cooperation is essential, and his involvement in the test should be outlined fully. During the first part of the test the patient is asked to relax in a dimly lit, quiet room with his eyes closed. This establishes his EEG baseline. Everyone has a unique set of brain waves. These change somewhat over long periods, but remain quite similar.

After he is used to the recording procedure and the EEG baseline is established, the hyperventilation segment of the test is begun. The patient is asked to breathe deeply and rapidly through his mouth for approximately three minutes while the EEG is being recorded. Hyperventilation often causes slight dizziness and tingling of the hands and feet, but these are transient sensations. After the hyperventilation EEG is obtained, the recording is continued to determine how soon the baseline is reestablished.

Many laboratories also use photic stimulation. A flickering light is focused on the patient while his eyes are closed and the EEG is recorded. The light may evoke abnormal discharges, especially seizure potentials.

If possible, drowsing and sleeping EEG runs are made. The patient is asked to try to sleep. If he can't, sleeping medication is given. Good patient preparation is most important during this portion of the examination. Drowsing and sleep EEG recordings done without medication may provide clues to brain dysfunction which might be masked by sleeping medication.

The quality of EEG recording can be enhanced by following this or a similar method of patient preparation. A demonstration by the EEG department can be helpful for personnel who are unfamiliar with this procedure. Adequate explanations of EEG and other diagnostic procedures provide a great measure of relief to any patient.

Section II
Some Common Neurological Disorders

Most people suffer an occasional headache, but when headaches are frequent occurrences or disrupt the person's life-style intervention may be necessary. The nurse can serve in a primary role for such clients. Seizures are less commonly seen in the general population, but can be disabling. Because seizures often are indicative of neurological disease, nurses must have a thorough understanding of their mechanism and treatment. The final two articles in this section concern the treatment and rehabilitation of persons with Parkinson's disease.

Vascular and Tension Headaches

LOIS M. HOSKINS

Headaches often have some basis in the client's lifestyle. Determining patterns and relationships can challenge the nurse.

"If one should search for the human ill which has manifested itself most widely during all times and among all people, there can be but little doubt that headache would attain this unenviable distinction"(1). Seventy percent of the people in the United States have headaches at some time; of this number, 10 to 12 percent seek medical help for their headaches. From September 1967 to September 1968, 6.1 million patient visits to physicians yielded a diagnosis of migraine, other forms of vascular headache, or tension headache, and during this period, persons being treated for headache had a total of nearly 5,300,000 days of restricted activity(2).

Chronic, recurring headaches can be classified in two categories. Ten percent of the patients treated by physicians have evidence of intracranial lesions, systemic disease, or psychotic states as a basis for their headaches. The remaining 90 percent have vascular headaches, muscle contraction (tension) headaches, or a combination of these two(2).

Any person with headache should have general physical and neurological examinations and laboratory tests. The outcome of these tests usually determines whether there is a serious organic cause for the headache, such as trauma, tumor, or subarachnoid hemorrhage. If there is none, treatment becomes a process of identifying the causes or triggering factors of the headache and successful methods for its treatment and pre-

---

MS. HOSKINS *(University of Iowa Hospital School of Nursing, Iowa City; B.S., Columbia Union College, Takoma Park, Md.; M.S.N., Catholic University, Washington, D.C.) is an assistant professor of medical-surgical nursing at Catholic University, Washington, D.C.*

vention. This can be a time-consuming process, and requires a trusting relationship between the parties involved. The magnitude and elusiveness of the problem, the time required to manage it, and the need for rapport make the treatment of headache ideally suited to the nurse, especially to a nurse in the primary care role.

The primary care nurse performs the initial assessment of the individual, and is responsible for his care and treatment. She collaborates with the physician or refers the client to other services as the need arises. Her goals are to deal with the immediate problem, prevent serious illness, and maintain or improve the client's health.

In working with the client, the nurse will use the nursing process, including assessment of the individual to identify his problems, planning and intervention to treat them, and evaluation.

ASSESSMENT

The initial patient information is obtained through conventional history taking, which includes the client's biographical data (age, sex, marital status, occupation, residence, economic status), his emotional and physical developmental status, his position in the family, the ages of other family members, and his past health history.

An elaborate history should be taken regarding his headache, including the following information:

Onset: At what age did the client first have headaches? What was happening in his life at the time? If possible, establish whether or not the onset coincided with a life crisis.

Frequency: How often do the headaches occur? Daily, weekly, bimonthly? At what time of day do they occur? On arising, in the afternoon, at night?

Duration: How long do the headaches last? Minutes, hours, days?

Nature of the pain: This is important in determining the cause of the headaches. Is the pain dull, aching, sharp, throbbing, mild, severe, unbearable? Is there a sense of fullness in the head, pressure behind the eyes, constricting bands, or tightness in the back of the neck? Determine what aggravates the pain. Lifting, bending, any kind of exertion? Or is the pain persistent and unremitting?

Location: Is the pain temporal, occipital, frontal, unilateral, bilateral, or generalized? Does it start in one area and move to another. Does it gradually encompass the whole head and neck?

Prodomal signs and symptoms: Establish whether or not the headaches come on suddenly or gradually, and whether there is a warning. Classical migraine headaches are typically preceded by an aura. Were there any visual disturbances, such as blurring or changes in light patterns? Some people experience paresthesias or other neurological signs. Was there a stuffiness in the nose, fullness in the head, or vague unrest prior to the headache?

Associated symptoms: Establish whether or not the client had any other physical symptoms at the time of the headache, such as nausea, vomiting, fatigue, chills, clamminess, weakness, swelling, or puffiness of the ankles or fingers.

Causes: Can the client ascribe any cause to the headache? Perhaps he had an emotional upset before its onset. Does the woman relate it to her menstrual cycle? Vascular headaches of a migraine nature may be caused by an antigen-antibody reaction or an allergic response(3). Therefore, the nurse notes any history of allergies. If the client has none, are there any relationships and patterns of precipitating factors, such as seasonal changes, foods eaten, or environmental allergens? If an undiagnosed allergy is suspected, the client should be referred to a physician for testing and treatment.

Family history: The majority of patients with migraine have a family history of migraine(4). Ask the patient if any relative has headaches, and if so, their nature and how the relative treats them.

Treatment: How does the client treat his headache? Does he take aspirin, narcotics, tranquilizers, sedatives? Can he continue moderate activity or must he go to bed? Does he usually lie down in a quiet, darkened room, or does he prefer to sit up? Does he apply cold or hot packs to the painful area? Does any of this give him relief?

Interviewing a client is not just a question-and-answer process. The nurse should begin her observations when she first meets the client and shakes his hand. What is his appearance? What is his color? Does he appear tired and exhausted? Is he well-groomed? Does he smile? Are his palms sweaty? Notice whether his responses to questions are short, reluc-

CHARACTERISTICS OF COMMON VASCULAR

Type of Headache	Onset	Frequency	Duration	Nature of Pain	Location
VASCULAR Classic Migraine	May begin at any age, usually adolescence.	Periodic and recurrent.	Usually 4-6 hours.	Usually severe.	Unilateral frontal, or temporal at onset, but may vary.
Common Migraine	May begin at any age. Gradual onset.	Episodic. Increase with life crisis.	Many hours to several days.	Usually starts slowly and builds throbbing aching pain. May awaken with severe headache.	Variable. May start unilaterally and spread.
Cluster Migraine	May start in early adulthood. Usually precipitated by vasodilators, alcohol, nitrites, histamine. Sudden onset.	Many attacks in quick succession over few days or weeks followed by remission which lasts for months.	Few minutes to few hours; usually 30-90 minutes.	Intense pain, boring, throbbing. Starts and stops suddenly.	Usually unilateral.
MUSCLE CONTRACTION (Tension)	Usually in adolescence. Associated with tension or anxiety. Gradual onset.	Varies with stress. Episodic.	Variable. Can be constant without treatment.	Dull, constant, tight band pressure. Non-pulsating. Varies in intensity.	Usually bilateral, but may be poorly defined. Involves neck, shoulders, occiput. May spread to frontal region.

tant, or lengthy. Does he attempt to intellectualize his problem? Observe his position and mannerisms. Does he fidget and squirm in the chair? Do his verbal responses correlate with his nonverbal ones?

The assessment will also include questions about, and physical examination of, the body's systems, with particular attention to any complaints the client voices. The client's blood pressure, and any changes in weight, vision, swelling, and urination patterns should be carefully assessed.

With this data base the nurse consults with the physician to determine what further diagnostic tests should be done to confirm or rule out a pathologic basis for the headaches. If there is no pathology, the client's

HEADACHES AND TENSION HEADACHES

Prodomal Signs and Symptoms	Associated Symptoms	Remarks
Transient visual field defects. Transient paresthesias, paralysis of an extremity, or confusion. These subside as pain begins.	Irritability, photophobia, nausea, vomiting, constipation or diarrhea, chills, tremors, pallor, sweating.	Hereditary incidence high. Following attack, often have feeling of well-being, unusual energy. Personality factors often contribute.
No striking prodome. May have changes in fluid balance. GI symptoms, vague psychic disturbances for several hours or days before onset of headache.	Nausea, vomiting, fatigue, chills, localized or general edema and diuresis, nasal stuffiness (autonomic disturbances).	Hereditary incidence high. Often relieved by pregnancy, illness. May be correlated with "let down" activities: "Weekend, Monday, menstrual, premenstrual, relaxation headache."
Uncommon.	Profuse watering and redness of conjunctiva, nasal stuffiness, increased perspiration, swelling of temporal vessels.	May be a family history of migraine. More common in older men. During remission, usual precipitants (alcohol) do not cause attack.
None.	Sustained contraction of neck and head muscles.	No familial history.

complaints can be compared to those listed in the chart to determine the type of headache he probably has.

PLANNING AND INTERVENTION

If the client has a vascular or muscle contraction headache, the nurse must decide on a plan of care for him. Her goals will be to alleviate his pain, establish the cause of triggering factors of the headaches, and to prevent or decrease their occurrence. Her plans will include methods for treatment, teaching, and further collection of data.

Medication may be prescribed for immediate relief of the client's pain.

Ergot alkaloids are the drugs of choice for treating vascular headaches of the migraine type. Their efficacy is often considered diagnostic of migraine. Diuretics have not proved successful, and the use of hormones has shown questionable results(4). In fact, oral contraceptives usually aggravate migraine(4).

If the client has migraine headaches, he should be instructed to take the medication at the onset of the attack. Although the exact physiological mechanisms involved in migraine are unknown, it is postulated that vasomotor changes in extracranial arteries cause the pain. The sequence is vasoconstriction, followed by vasodilatation, and then edema of these arteries(5). Medication must be taken well before the edema phase. Also, the client should determine the most effective initial dosage and always take that amount at the onset of a headache. He should then repeat the dosage as ordered until maximum relief is obtained.

Clients who have muscle contraction headaches can lessen their severity by taking analgesics or muscle relaxants at the onset. Both types of headache can be relieved somewhat if the person retires to a quiet, darkened room. The person with vascular headache may choose to sit rather than lie down. Cold packs may relieve or aggravate a vascular headache; pressure applied to the temporal and carotid arteries may be helpful.

Persons who cannot take ergotamine preparations because of severe side effects or contraindications may get relief from other drugs. Aspirin may be taken alone or in combination with non-narcotic analgesics, such as phenacetin, acetaminophen, or propoxyphene (Darvon). Codeine may also be used. Meperidine and morphine are not recommended because of their dependence liability. Taking a mild sedative or relaxant, such as phenobarbital or meprobamate, with an analgesic may help to reduce anxiety, promote rest, and alter the reaction to pain. Various combinations of analgesics and sedatives, muscle relaxants, or caffeine are available commercially. The effectiveness of any of these drugs varies with the individual and the circumstances of the headache.

Because pregnant women cannot take the ergot derivatives, some of the above medications may be prescribed, but only with extra caution during the first trimester. Interestingly enough, migraine attacks usually disappear completely after the first few months of pregnancy. If headaches reappear in the last trimester, the client should be assessed for possible toxemia.

Continued treatment is aimed at establishing the cause of the client's headache. To do this, a continuing assessment and reassessment of his personality, habits, and daily activities must be undertaken.

Some information may be obtained during the initial interview. The

DRUGS FOR VASCULAR MIGRAINE HEADACHES

Drug	Dosage	Action	Side Effects	Comments
Ergotamine tartrate (1) Orally or sublingually	2-4mg. at start of attack, followed by 1-2mg. every hour until headache is relieved or 10mg. of drug have been taken.	Constricts cerebral blood vessels, reducing cerebral blood flow.	Nausea, vomiting, epigastric discomfort, muscle pains in extremities, numbness and tingling in extremities, transient bradycardia or tachycardia, localized edema, and itching.	Important to use medication at onset of headache. Do not take during pregnancy (an oxytocic). Do not take in presence of sepsis or vascular, kidney, or liver diseases. Habituation may lead to rebound reaction and further headache. Dependency may develop if used daily (usually by people with underlying depression).
(2) Rectally	2-4mg. at onset, followed by 2 mg. every hour until headache is relieved or 8mg. have been taken.			
(3) Subcutaneously or intramuscularly	0.25 to 0.5mg. at onset. Dose may be repeated hourly up to 1mg. in 24 hours.			
(4) Intravenously (rarely)	0.25mg. at onset; no more than 0.5mg. in 24 hours.			
Ergotamine with caffeine	Varies with commercial preparation used.	Caffeine constricts cerebral blood vessels. This enhances action of ergot alkaloids and may decrease dosage of ergot needed.	Same as ergotamine	Same as ergotamine
Ergotamine with caffeine, a sedative (phenobarbital), and an antispasmodic (belladonna)	Varies with commercial preparation used.	Vasoconstriction, sedation, reduces spasm.	Same as ergotamine, plus dryness of mucous membranes, drowsiness.	Same as ergotamine. Contraindicated in persons with glaucoma.
Dihydroergotamine (D.H.E.)	1mg. IM at onset of headache. May be repeated in 1 hr. with limit of 2mg. Can be given I.V. to maximum of 2mg.	Vasoconstriction	Same as ergotamine.	Same as ergotamine.
Methysergide Maleate (Sansert)	2mg. 3 to 4 times daily.	Prophylactic. Weak vasoconstriction. Serotonin antagonist. Exact action unknown.	Frequently encountered. Abdominal discomfort, muscle cramps, edema, paresthesias of extremities, depression. Fibrotic complications occasionally develop with long term therapy, including retroperitoneal fibrosis and pleuropulmonary and cardiac fibrosis.	Should only be used in persons whose headaches are frequent and disabling. Close medical supervision needed.

Based on information from Friedman's "Drug Treatment of Migraine," pp. 96-103 (5), and Goodman and Gilman's *Pharmacologic Basis of Therapeutics*, 1970, pp. 900-905.

nurse uses judgment in determining how and when to elicit details. If the client presents himself initially with a headache and is anxious, his immediate needs should be met and lengthy assessment postponed. Also, meeting the client several times, visiting him at home, and talking with his family can give the nurse additional opportunities to establish rapport with him and make her own observations.

All behavior has a purpose and the nurse seeks to determine what purpose, if any, the client's headache serves. Internal conflicts lead to anxiety and anxiety may be manifested through the headaches. Migraine sufferers are often characterized as being perfectionistic, rigid, compulsive, extremely sensitive, and conscientious. They have been described as ambitious, hard-driving people who work themselves into exhaustion and then develop a headache that allows them to relax and rebuild their energy stores. They may come from families where thoughts, feelings, and emotions are not expressed. They may set high standards and feel guilt if they are compromised(6). The individual with muscle contraction headaches responds to stress with increased anxiety and tension. Both groups are likely to repress hostility and anger. Psychosexual conflicts may be present. The headaches may hide a more serious emotional disorder or they may serve purposes of secondary gain(6).

For example, one teen-ager's headaches began when she was preparing for an exam. She was a straight "A" student who excelled on written exams. On this occasion each student was to be questioned orally in front of the class. An hour before the exam she had a visual aura, developed a severe headache with nausea and vomiting, and had to go home. She has had a history of migraine since that time.

The nurse attempts to gain more insight into her client's personality characteristics. It is easy to fall into the trap of stereotyping clients as having a "migraine personality." Everyone must be treated as an individual. Many of us have the qualities described but rarely have headaches; others have headaches without having these traits.

The following questions may help determine a client's personality characteristics. The questions should be open-ended and the client should be given time to elaborate on his answers.

Work habits: Does he like perfection in all of his work? Does he work overtime without compensation? Do his co-workers share these attributes? Does he have a schedule for each day's activities? If so, can it be changed at the last minute?

Aspirations: What are his goals? What does he think of himself? How does he respond to criticism? Probably of greater importance is the person's ability to understand when he is under stress and how to manage it. Somatic complaints often arise from repressed hostility.

Family relationships: Is he physically demonstrative to his spouse, children, and parents? Is he satisfied with his sexual relationships? Does he talk about sex with his wife? Who is "boss" in the family? How is punishment decided on and meted out? How does his family react to his headaches?

Reactions to stress: Try to learn the client's coping mechanisms. In a verbal disagreement does he close up or does he talk it out? Does he remain upset for several days following a minor disagreement?

Relaxation: Identify the time he spends relaxing and the nature of his hobbies. Does the family share his interests?

The next step in implementation is to have the client keep a calendar of his daily activities and his headaches, to determine whether there is a relationship between the two. The client may be reluctant to do this, but if his headaches are being relieved somewhat and he has confidence in the nurse he will probably give it a try. He should record business, social, and home activities, and note whether these were usual or unusual and how he felt about them. Maybe he hates the way his wife looks every morning. He should note how he slept each night to determine if he has insomnia and, if so, when it occurs. How much sleep does he think he needs? He should list what he eats, and describe any eating binges or unusual food cravings. Does he drink alcohol? When and how much? He should note the physical exercise or relaxation he gets each day. Women should observe somatic changes, such as a vaginal discharge, swollen, tender breasts, or bloaty feeling. It is important to describe the mood of the day. Was he irritable, snappy, happy, depressed? Was the client's mood appropriate for the circumstances?

On his headache calendar he should record the onset, duration, location, severity, prodomes, and associated symptoms of each headache he had. He should record its treatment to determine what drugs and related measures are effective. One problem here is that all headaches are not the same and so all do not respond to the same therapy. Migraine sufferers also have tension headaches, and *vice versa.*

Using this information, nurse and client should be able to determine his body rhythm, identify any patterns of recurring behavior, and recognize triggering factors. These may be fatigue, hunger, alcohol, bright lights, stress, menstruation, or climatic changes. In some people, specific situations provoke attacks; in others, it is an accumulation or variety of circumstances.

One woman found that she invariably became tense and eventually hostile toward her neighbors when they gathered for their morning coffee *klatsch*. She wanted to join them but she did not have her morning work done and would not allow herself this time off until she had completed her work. Eventually her self-punishment provoked a headache.

Another man worked very hard at the office all week and looked forward to sleeping late and doing nothing on the weekend. He invariably woke up every Saturday with a stuffy nose and severe headache.

Once the psychodynamics of the headache are clarified, keeping the calendar and seeing the relationships may be enough to help the client decide he must make some changes in his activities and life-style.

If the person with chronic headaches seems more tired at a particular time of the month, he should not schedule any major activity for that period. If the woman knows that she is more irritable and likely to have headaches during the middle and end of her menstrual cycle, she can plan accordingly.

The family is included in any plan of care. They will have been asked to contribute to the assessment and now may need to know the relationships of various activities to the client's headaches. It may be difficult for them to understand the guilt feelings that can occur about completing tasks, doing a good job, being a good mother, father, wife, or husband. Yet this understanding may help the person to overcome his guilt feelings and thus relieve his headaches.

Many headaches may be brought on by pushing oneself. While it is easy to tell a client to "take it easy," this may upset him and lead to even more headaches. It is more important to help him understand his problems, learn about his body, realize when pressures are accumulating, and develop a pattern of taking little moments of relaxation as a relief valve.

For the client who has weekend or let-down headaches, the nurse may suggest that he arise at the same time and in the same fashion as he does on weekdays, and plan an activity for the day. It also helps people who awaken with a stuffy feeling to elevate the head of the bed several inches.

If the client has conflicts which he prefers not to recognize or which may cause serious psychological problems if they are exposed, the nurse collaborates with a psychiatrist in the treatment.

Some persons are reluctant to change their life-style because they have heard that they will outgrow their headaches. This is not necessarily true. Individual migraine histories vary considerably. Some people develop headaches in childhood and have them throughout their lives; others start having headaches during puberty and stop having them after menopause. Some people are headache free for years and then experience recurrence, and others note alterations in the frequency and severity of their headaches. Classical migraine is more apt to disappear with age than common migraine. Because attacks usually occur with life crises, if an individual has learned to cope effectively with these crises as he grows older, his headaches may decrease.

EVALUATION

The final step in the nursing process is evaluation. Has the headache pain been alleviated? Have the cause and triggering factors been established? Has the frequency been reduced? Evaluation is a continuing process. To be meaningful, it must consist of further assessment, planning, and revision to identify possible triggering factors and to establish the best methods of treatment and prevention.

Perhaps the greatest help will be the nurse herself. She must listen to the client, be able to empathize with him, and yet be intellectually and emotionally honest in analyzing his situation. The client may be unable or not care to change his patterns and habits, but if he can confide his thoughts and feelings to someone this may provide enough of an outlet to decrease his headaches. If he does undertake changing some of his living patterns, she may give him the support he needs. In her primary care role she will continue to help him achieve and maintain better health and so, hopefully, ease the pain in his head.

REFERENCES

1. RILEY, H. A. *Migraine. Bull.Neurol.Inst.* (New York) 2:429-544, Nov. 1932
2. HURLEY, F. E. *Practical Management of Headache in Office Practice.* Paper presented at Scientific Exhibit, Chicago Medical Society, Mar. 2-5, 1969.
3. SHAPIRO, R. S. Allergic headache. IN *Handbook of Clinical Neurology. Volume 5. Headaches and Cranial Neuralgias,* ed. by P. J. Vinken and G. W. Bruyn, New York, American Elsevier, 1968, pp. 234-237.
4. FRIEDMAN, A. P. Current concepts in the diagnosis and treatment of chronic recurring headache. *Med.Clin.NorthAm.* 56:1261-1269, Nov. 1962.
5. ———. Migraine, pathophysiology and pathogenesis. IN *Handbook of Clinical Neurology. Volume 5. Headaches and Cranial Neuralgias,* ed. by P. J. Vinken and G. W. Bruyn, New York, American Elsevier, 1968, pp. 37-44.
6. BOAG, T. J. Psychogenic headache. IN *Handbook of Clinical Neurology. Volume 5. Headaches and Cranial Neuralgias,* ed. by P. J. Vinken and G. W. Bruyn. New York, American Elsevier, 1968, pp. 247-257.

Epilepsy: A Controllable Disease
Classification and Diagnosis of Seizures

MARGARET AULD BRUYA • ROSE HOMAN BOLIN

A new classification of seizure activity facilitates better understanding of the pathophysiology.

A seizure is not a disease; it is a symptom of a disease. When "seizure" is mentioned, one generally thinks of loss of consciousness, violent jerking movements, and foaming at the mouth—the behavior observed when a person has a grand mal seizure.

This picture is incomplete, for not all seizures are visible. There are gradations of seizures, as well as different types and causes. Most physicians define a seizure as a transitory disturbance in consciousness or in motor, sensory, or autonomic function that is due to uncontrolled electrical discharges in the brain.

Over the years many words have been used to describe a seizure, among them, spell, fit, and attack. *Convulsion* is more specific and describes a seizure manifested by jerking movements of the entire body. *Seizure* is the English translation of the Greek word *epilepsia* (to take or seize), and the two terms are used synonymously.

If a specific brain lesion is the cause of the seizure, the condition may be called symptomatic epilepsy. Seizures may be a symptom, for example, of cerebral trauma, intracranial tumor or infections, cerebral vascular disease, and drug toxicity or withdrawal.

If neurological examination does not pinpoint the cause of the sei-

---

MARGARET AULD BRUYA, *R.N., M.N., is an assistant professor, Department of Nursing, Rhode Island College. She was an assistant professor in the Department of Physiological Nursing at the University of Washington, Seattle when this article was written.* ROSE HOMAN BOLIN, *R.N., M.A., is an instructor, Department of Physiological Nursing, University of Washington.*

zures, the condition is labeled *idiopathic epilepsy*. Idiopathic epilepsy is most frequently identified before puberty and is associated with a familial tendency. The practice of classifying epilepsy as idiopathic or symptomatic has declined in recent years.

Seizure disorders also may be viewed as acute or chronic. *Acute epilepsy* usually is related to such metabolic disorders as hypocalcemia, hypoglycemia, or drug withdrawal. In *chronic epilepsy*, seizures tend to recur and the primary defect is in the brain. The episodes do not stem from an extracerebral cause or from a transient insult(1). Most physicians restrict the diagnosis of epilepsy to this recurring disorder, and we will use the term "epilepsy" in this sense.

Regardless of the type of seizure, the basic cause is the same: abnormal and excessive electrical discharges from the brain. The electrical abnormality may arise from the central areas of the brain and immediately affect consciousness, or it may be restricted to one part of the cortex and produce only signs and symptoms characteristic of that anatomical focus. In a third type of seizure the electrical abnormality may begin in a localized area of the cortex, spread to normal brain tissue, and, if sufficiently extensive, activate the central brain, which would then result in loss of consciousness and tonic-clonic motions.

Seizure activity appears to be initiated by a group of abnormal cells referred to as the *epileptogenic focus*. What causes these epileptic neurons to be hyperexcitable is not known. An epileptogenic focus may remain quiescent over a period of time, discharging intermittently but restrained from spreading by normal inhibitory mechanisms. Such a focus does not produce signs and symptoms, but it may be revealed by the electroencephalogram (EEG). Physiological changes may trigger the focus or facilitate the spread of seizure activity to normal tissue. Such precipitating factors include abnormal blood sugar levels; changes in blood gas tensions, plasma pH, or serum osmolality; electrolyte imbalances or endocrine changes; fatigue or emotional stress; and some nutritional deficiencies. Thus, an otherwise healthy person may experience seizure activity if he has an acute alteration of his body chemistries.

The many different terms to describe epilepsy and the systems to classify it can be confusing. These have included attempts to classify epilepsy according to the nature of the seizure, its underlying cause, the type of EEG changes, or the patient's response to therapy.

Unfortunately, none of these classifications has been universally accepted. We have found a modification of Schmidt's and Wilder's system most useful(2). It classifies epilepsy according to the clinical form of the seizure, a system that aids in organizing and understanding the pathophysiology and inferred nursing care.

With this classification, seizures are categorized as generalized, partial, or miscellaneous. Generalized and partial seizures are seen most commonly.

GENERALIZED SEIZURES

Generalized seizures without focal onset seem to arise in the reticular formation of the brain stem and have a diffuse, nonspecific influence on cerebral function. Characteristically, the patient reports no aura or warning and loses consciousness at the onset. The seizures may occur at any time of the day or night, and may recur from minutes to hours to years apart, without seasonal variation.

Most patients in this group first experience seizures in childhood, and 90 percent develop symptoms before age 20. Most patients have no organic disease and their seizures may have a hereditary basis. Generalized seizures occurring after the age of 20 are most likely due to other pathology, such as a brain tumor, vascular abnormality, or cerebral trauma. More specifically, these are usually focal seizures that are secondarily generalized, a type of seizure activity to be discussed later.

GRAND MAL Of the generalized seizures without focal onset, the grand mal is the most dramatic. No matter what a person is doing at the onset, he immediately loses consciousness and, if standing, falls to the floor. It is important for the nurse to ascertain if the person had any symptoms before losing consciousness. Formerly, grand mal seizures were thought to be preceded by an aura. An aura does not occur with a true grand mal seizure, but is associated with secondary generalization, a type of partial seizure(3).

Loss of consciousness occurs immediately and is due to the electrical discharges that overwhelm the brain's subcortical center, which is primarily responsible for alertness. Within seconds the tonic phase of the seizure begins and lasts approximately 10 to 20 seconds. Symmetrical involvement of all skeletal muscles is observed. The patient's body stiffens; his arms usually flex; and his legs, head, and neck extend. His jaws clamp shut and the thoracic abdominal muscles contract, forcing air across tightly closed vocal cords and producing the "epileptic cry," which may last from 2 to 12 seconds. Because he does not breathe during this time, he becomes cyanotic. Due to the stimulation of the autonomic nervous system, salivation increases and secretions collect in the throat.

The patient then enters the clonic phase, lasting about 30 seconds. The tonic rigidity becomes less pronounced and violent jerking motions of his entire body begin. During this time, he may foam at the mouth as he breathes through the accumulated oropharyngeal secretions, and the bladder may empty as the sphincter relaxes. The jerking movements gradually diminish in intensity, occur at longer intervals, and finally cease.

In the postictal state, the patient appears to relax but complete muscle relaxation and return of autonomic function do not occur immediately. The patient cannot be easily aroused, but may awaken in four to five minutes in a state of confusion. Left alone, he normally sleeps for several hours. He often awakens fully conscious but feels very tired, complains of sore muscles and a headache, and is usually amnesic for the total event.

Most grand mal seizures last only a few minutes. If they do not stop spontaneously or the patient passes from one seizure to another without regaining consciousness, he is said to be in *status epilepticus*. If not interrupted, such successive grand mal seizures lead to respiratory failure and death.

PETIT MAL EPILEPSY is a type of generalized seizure that may go unrecognized because the person's behavior changes very little. Sometimes the affected person's only clue that he has had an attack is that he has to reorient himself to his previous activity. Children have been known to ride bicycles during petit mal epilepsy without injury, because they maintained postural control.

Petit mal almost always begins in early childhood and, in many patients, stops at puberty. Less than 50 percent of children with petit mal develop grand mal seizures. Adult onset of petit mal is unusual and probably represents childhood petit mal that went unrecognized until adulthood. Some adults who have "petit mal" symptoms actually have another type of seizure or they may have a behavioral disorder that mimics a neurological condition.

Hyperventilation, hypoglycemia, emotional and physiological stresses, and normal fatigue and sleepiness can precipitate petit mal seizures. As many as 50 to 100 episodes per day have been reported and it is likely that some children have many more episodes.

MYOCLONIC SEIZURES are characterized by sudden, brief, muscular contractions, occurring singly or repetitively, that may or may not be symmetrical. Diffuse brain involvement is noted on the EEG. The myoclonic jerk (arms jerk together and upward, the trunk flexes) may be severe enough to throw the patient to the ground or off his bed. Myoclonic seizures may be part of many neurological syndromes and do not necessarily signify a deteriorating disease.

AKINETIC SEIZURES are manifested by a sudden loss of muscle tone and postural control, and the patient may fall to the floor. Because he does not have postural reflexes and therefore does not put out his hand to break the fall, he can incur a head or shoulder injury. The EEG may be diffusely abnormal. Akinetic seizures often do not respond to any therapy and, like other primary generalized seizures, have no aura. Consequently, patients may be instructed to wear football helmets for cranial protection.

The patient who has either myoclonic or akinetic seizures usually does not bite his tongue or become incontinent. Whether unconsciousness occurs is debatable since both types of seizure occur so quickly and recovery is so rapid. Akinetic seizures have a hereditary link and normally appear before age 15.

PARTIAL OR FOCAL SEIZURES

A partial or focal seizure is due to abnormal electrical discharges in a localized part of the cortex. The irritating focus of such a seizure is secondary to an underlying condition that damages brain tissue.

Congenital anomalies or birth injury are frequent causes of focal seizures in children. With increasing age, there is a greater probability that such acquired conditions as a brain tumor or trauma are responsible.

Focal seizures may arise from any part of the cortex, but the frontal, parietal, and temporal lobes are most often affected. The clinical manifestation of the seizure is closely correlated to the affected site. For example, seizures originating in the motor strip of the cortex characteristically produce clonic movements of a limb or part of a limb. Most frequently the onset of a motor seizure is seen in the hand and face, less commonly in the trunk or leg. These movements may last 20 to 30 seconds with no alteration in the patient's level of consciousness.

If the seizure begins in the sensory cortex, numbness and tingling will be experienced in the affected part of the body. Auditory, vestibular, and visual seizures reflect a lesion or irritation in the corresponding part of the brain.

PARTIAL SEIZURES with complex symptomatology involve more organized and higher level cerebral function, such as affect, memory, and cognition, in addition to sensory and motor function. Because the seizure has behavioral manifestations as well as patterned motor movements, it is often called a psychomotor seizure. The temporal lobe is the most common source, so seizures of this type are also frequently termed temporal lobe epilepsy.

CLASSIFICATION OF SEIZURES

GENERALIZED SEIZURES WITHOUT FOCAL ONSET

    grand mal

    petit mal

    myoclonic seizures

    akinetic seizures

PARTIAL OR FOCAL SEIZURES, WITH OR WITHOUT GENERALIZATION

    partial or focal seizures
      motor seizures
      sensory seizures

    partial seizures with complex symptomatology—psychomotor or temporal lobe epilepsy
      automatisms
      visceral and autonomic, including olfactory and gustatory
      psychic (illusory, hallucinatory)
      affective symptoms

MISCELLANEOUS

    erratic seizures with inconsistent or changing patterns

    unclassified because of inadequate or incomplete information

    epileptic syndromes (classified separately because of the complex inter-relationship between the seizures and the neurological disease of which they may be the major symptom, such as hereditary myoclonus epilepsy and infantile myoclonic encephalopathy)

    other seizures of childhood, including febrile seizures

This table is a modification of the classification proposed by Schmidt and Wilder in *Epilepsy—A Clinical Textbook,* Philadelphia. F. A. Davis Company, 1968, p. 7.

Psychomotor seizures comprise about one third of the chronic seizure disorders, and are more common in adults than children. They are manifested in various ways, ranging from a brief loss of consciousness to longer episodes of purposeless activity.

The most frequent sensation at the beginning of a psychomotor seizure is a strange feeling in the pit of the stomach which rises toward the throat. At the same time the patient may notice an unpleasant odor or hear strange noises, such as the ringing of bells. Because some aspects of memory are stored in the temporal lobe, memory disturbances are often a component of the psychomotor seizure. Patients sometimes experience *déjà vu*—they suddenly relive vivid scenes from the past or have intense feelings of familiarity while in strange environments. *Déjà vu* also occurs in people without epilepsy when exhausted or under emotional stress. Other mental symptoms of psychomotor seizures include a distorted perception of time and self, and strong emotions, such as fear or anxiety.

The motor component of the psychomotor seizure varies considerably from person to person and usually consists of patterned automatic motor movements. Some psychomotor seizures last four to five minutes. In the postictal period, confusion and amnesia usually are present and may be prolonged.

Because of the wide variety of behavioral manifestations associated with a psychomotor seizure, it is often difficult to determine whether they are related to an epileptic seizure or a nonepileptic behavioral disturbance. An abnormality in the EEG over the temporal lobe reinforces the diagnosis of psychomotor seizure disorder. Because the abnormal discharges are sometimes seen during sleep, an EEG is often performed at this time. If the diagnosis is still uncertain, the patient may be placed on antiepileptic medication as a therapeutic trial. A favorable reponse to medication strengthens the probability of temporal lobe epilepsy.

SECONDARY GENERALIZATION Partial or focal seizures may spread to other parts of the brain and become generalized convulsive episodes or major motor seizures. This process, called secondary generalization, is recognized as a separate entity.

Any focal seizure can send abnormal impulses to the central brain, which, in turn, may discharge electrical impulses of its own and produce a generalized convulsive seizure. Thus, the symptoms of the focal seizure —motor, sensory, or psychic—precede the generalized seizure. The aura is not a symptom that heralds the onset of a seizure, but is the early stages of the attack itself(4).

The symptoms of the focal disturbance provide an important diagnostic clue to the location of the underlying brain lesion. Any adult who has a generalized convulsive seizure should be examined for the presence of a focal abnormality because a true grand mal seizure disorder rarely develops after puberty.

A good example of a focal seizure with secondary generalization is the "Jacksonian march." This begins with localized clonic motions of the hand, foot, or face. As the electrical impulses spread to contiguous regions of the cortex, the clonic movements "march" to the body parts activated by those regions. Thus, a seizure beginning in the hand will spread to the arm and face, then down the leg to the foot. If the electrical discharges spread to the center of the brain, a generalized convulsive seizure and loss of consciousness result. Although the Jacksonian seizure has been given much attention in the literature, it is rarely seen.

MISCELLANEOUS SEIZURES

Of the seizures classified as miscellaneous, the febrile seizure of childhood causes the most concern and misconceptions. Some experts question the need for a thorough neurological workup when a child has been otherwise healthy and has no history of epileptic seizures or head trauma. But because a febrile seizure *may* be a generalized seizure disorder heralded or precipitated by a fever, arriving at a diagnosis can be more complex.

Febrile seizures typically occur when a child is between six months and four years old. The generalized seizure is brief, normally less than five minutes, and occurs only when the child had a high temperature. The seizure is similar to the grand mal type, and has no focal onset. A child with a focal-onset seizure that is associated with a fever and an abnormal EEG does not have a true febrile seizure disorder; he or she should be evaluated further.

Some families seem prone to have children with febrile seizures so the question of familial disposition is important in the diagnostic workup. An EEG taken 24 to 48 hours after a suspected febrile seizure should be normal.

As the central nervous system matures, febrile seizure activity diminishes and, by the time a child is six, he should have outgrown his tendency.

DIAGNOSIS OF SEIZURES DISORDERS

The medical and nursing assessment essential in determining the type of seizure disorder rests primarily on skilled observation, knowledge of the neurological system, and judicious use of diagnostic examinations.

A complete, accurate, and detailed history should be obtained from the most reliable and knowledgeable person. For pediatric patients, the past medical history should include information about the prenatal, delivery, and immediate postnatal periods, and about previous accidents or illnesses.

Episodes of altered consciousness should be explored, whether the patient is an adult or child. Seizures may be caused by acute alcoholism or by withdrawal from some drugs, particularly barbiturates and amphetamines, so the patient should be questioned about these possibilities.

The examiner can help a patient recall the seizure by asking about the presence of any sensation, odd feeling, or other detail he can remember. Descriptions of a seizure as seen by friends, school teachers, fellow workers, and family members may help localize a lesion otherwise thought to be a generalized seizure disorder, and can be particularly useful in establishing the person's diagnosis. Ideally, the seizure should be witnessed by a skilled observer.

The physical examination is intended to identify and localize the disorder of the nervous system. If the physical examination does not disclose a neurological basis for the seizures, the patient will need additional testing to determine if other physiological or emotional problems are causing the seizures.

Most of the diagnostic examinations cause little discomfort, but each should be explained to the patient. A person with a seizure disorder already is frightened because his symptoms threaten his ability to control his own behavior, so any control that he has been able to develop should be supported.

The diagnostic techniques include the noninvasive—x-ray including axial tomograms, electroencephalogram (EEG), echoencephalogram (ECHO), and brain scan—and the invasive—lumbar puncture, and tests that use contrast media, such as the arteriogram and pneumoencephalogram (PEG).

Skull x-rays are useful for the evaluation of increased intracranial pressure and for showing abnormal intracranial calcifications. Computerized axial tomograms identify benign conditions such as abscesses, cysts, and vascular abnormalities, and precisely define and localize malignant lesions. Data obtained from a brain scan helps to locate the site of focal lesions. The ECHO is helpful in evaluating mass brain lesions that displace midline structures.

The EEG, although not infallible, is the most useful diagnostic tool in the evaluation of seizure disorders. Electrical potential generated in living tissue can be measured and recorded on paper with the aid of electrodes placed over the cranium. Several EEGs may be done under varying conditions: with the patient sleeping, awake, awake with provocative stimulation (flashing lights or sounds), and hyperventilating. These conditions elicit abnormal electrical changes and, thus, changes in the EEG. Although the EEG is a helpful adjunct to the diagnosis, it may be inconclusive. Ten percent of patients who have had grand mal seizures have normal EEG tracings, and as many normal people have somewhat abnormal readings(5).

Invasive techniques are more distressing to the patient but rarely present a real danger to his health. The lumbar puncture yields information about possible infection or trauma and cerebrospinal fluid pressure. Arteriograms and PEGs help delineate vascular malformations and brain tumors.

Seizure disorders have been known for centuries, and we have come a long way from the times when the victim of "falling sickness" was thought to be possessed by the devil. With greater knowledge of its different manifestations and with rational therapy the modern epileptic is likely to have fewer seizures and to endure fewer indignities than he did in the past.

Drug Therapy and Nursing Care

Myth and social discrimination still surround the diagnosis of epilepsy.

As early as 2080 B.C., the Code of Hammurabi included rules about the marriage of epileptic persons and the validity of their court testimony. Hippocrates was the first to consider epilepsy a disease of the brain and in his monograph "On the Sacred Disease" attacked the superstition and magic that surrounded it(6).

In the 1850s an English physician, Sir Charles Locock, discovered almost by accident that bromide would control seizure activity in some epileptic patients. This remained the only known antiepileptic medication for 60 years.

In 1873 John Hughlings Jackson wrote the classical physiological definition of epilepsy, when he stated that seizures are "occasional, sudden, excessive, rapid, and local discharges of grey matter"(7).

Unfortunately, in some people, bromide therapy caused mental sluggishness, which prompted the association of epilepsy with low intelligence. During the late period of bromide therapy, many statutes were enacted that curtailed the rights of epileptics, by restricting their marriage or requiring sterilization. The typical medical view of epilepsy was that "the etiology of seizures was unknown, seizures were incurable, the condition was accompanied by progressive mental deterioration, and progeny of epileptics were likely to have seizures"(8).

In 1912 phenobarbital was found to reduce seizure activity without producing as much mental sluggishness as bromide. However, it was not until the discovery of phenytoin (Dilantin)[1] in 1938 that seizure control improved dramatically. At the same time electroencephalography came into widespread use and the diagnosis and treatment of epilepsy advanced rapidly. Thus, effective treatment of epilepsy is a recent development, which may account for lagging social attitudes regarding this disease. Experimentation with biofeedback and cerebellar stimulation in the last decade may open new avenues of therapy in the future.[2]

SEIZURE CONTROL

Epilepsy cannot be cured, but for most patients partial or complete control is possible with antiepileptic drugs. These are believed to act mainly by reducing the responsiveness of normal neurons to the periodic, sudden, high frequency nerve impulses originating from the epileptogenic focus. The regular use of antiepileptic medications results in significant seizure control in 70 to 80 percent of all patients with recurring seizures(9).

Phenytoin and phenobarbital are the drugs most commonly used for both generalized and partial seizure disorders. Another frequent combination is phenytoin and primidone (Mysoline). For the occasional patient who does not respond to the more common antiepileptics or who develops side effects from them, alternative drugs may be prescribed (see p. 47).

Petit mal seizures usually do not respond to the medications that control other generalized seizures. Ethosuximide (Zarontin) often is the drug of choice. Patients suffering from both petit mal and grand mal or psychomotor seizures need ethosuximide and one or more of the medications used to treat the second seizure disorder.

Another mode of therapy for petit mal epilepsy has been the ketogenic diet, which is high in fats and low in carbohydrates. This diet produces a mild metabolic acidosis—a shift in metabolism that makes the patient less prone to seizures. Because of the difficulty in adhering to this diet and the high degree of effectiveness of ethosuximide, the ketogenic diet

---

[1] Phenytoin is the new generic name for diphenylhydantoin (Dilantin).

[2] For information about cerebellar stimulation and biofeedback, see "Cerebellar Stimulation: Pacing the Brain," p. 101, and "Clinical Biofeedback," p. 2008, Nov. 1975, *AJN*.

ANTIEPILEPTIC DRUGS

Drugs of Choice	Indications	Usual adult maintenance dose, mg./day and (dose range)	Desirable blood concentration micrograms/ml.	Side effects and adverse reactions
phenytoin—new generic name for diphenylhydantoin (Dilantin)	generalized convulsive seizures, all forms of partial seizures; often in combination with primidone and/or phenobarbital	300 (200-600)	15-25	drowsiness, gastric distress, gingival hyperplasia, rash, megaloblastic anemia, ataxia, diplopia, fever, hirsuitism
phenobarbital (Luminal)	generalized convulsive seizures, all forms of partial seizures; often in combination with phenytoin	90 (60-400)	10-30	drowsiness, rash, ataxia
primidone (Mysoline)	generalized convulsive seizures, all forms of partial seizures; often in combination with phdnytoin and/or phenobarbital	750 (500-1500)	5-15	drowsiness, dizziness, rash, megaloblastic anemia, ataxia, diplopia, nystagmus
ethosuximide (Zarontin)	generalized nonconvulsive seizures, especially petit mal; used in mixed seizure states with phenytoin	750 (500-2000)	30-100	gastric distress, nausea, vomiting, anorexia, dermatitis, drowsiness, dizziness, blood dyscrasias
Alternative drugs				
carbamazepine (Tegretol)	generalized convulsive seizures, partial seizures, especially psychomotor; also used for treatment of trigeminal neuralgia	800 (600-1600)	3-6	headache, drowsiness, dizziness, feelings of inhibition, gait disturbances, blood dyscrasias
mephenytoin (Mesantoin)	generalized convulsive seizures, all forms of partial seizures	300 (300-800)		drowsiness, rash, blood dyscrasias
mephobarbital (Mebaral)	same as phenobarbital			drowsiness, irritability, rash
trimethadione (Tridione)	generalized nonconvulsive seizures—petit mal, myoclonic and akinetic; often used with phenytoin and phenobarbital	900 (900-2400)	600-800	drowsiness, gastric distress, rash hemeralopia, blood dyscrasias, nephrosis
paramethadione (Paradione)	generalized nonconvulsive seizures, especially petit mal; sometimes useful for psychomotor seizures	900 (900-2400)		gastric distress, rash, photophobia, blood dyscrasias
methsuximide (Celontin)	generalized nonconvulsive seizures, especially petit mal; sometimes useful for psychomotor seizures	900 (600-1200)		drowsiness, headaches, anorexia, blood dyscrasias, ataxia
phensuximide (Milontin)	generalized nonconvulsive seizures, sometimes useful for psychomotor seizures	1500 (1000-4000)		dizziness, hematuria, nausea, rash
phenacemide (Phenurone)	only used in resistant cases because of toxicity; all types of seizures, especially psychomotor	3000 (1000-6000)		liver damage, psychotic behavior, nausea, rash
acetazolamide (Diamox)	sometimes useful for petit mal seizures; in all seizure disorders as an adjuvant to control seizures related to menstrual cycle	750 (500-100)		anorexia, dizziness, drowsiness
detroamphetamine sulfate (Dexedrine)	used with some antiepileptics to counteract sedative effects; some therapeutic effect in petit mal	(15-30)		anorexia, irritability, insomnia

now is reserved for patients who do not respond to drug therapy.

Temporal lobe seizures are the most difficult to control. Patients may require phenytoin, phenobarbital, and primidone in full therapeutic doses. These medications control seizures significantly in 50 to 60 percent of cases(10). Surgical excision of a portion of the temporal lobe may be considered for patients who do not respond to medical management and who have a localized lesion as identified by EEG tracings. In carefully selected patients, such surgery reduces or eliminates seizure activity and improves mental symptoms.

Awareness of the many side effects associated with antiepileptic medications is important for all team members caring for people with epilepsy. Drowsiness may occur with all four drugs of choice, particularly in the first days of dosage adjustment. A rash or generalized dermatitis is another side effect common to all of these drugs. During the first days of its administration, phenytoin may cause stomach upset; this can be relieved by taking the medication with meals.

A distressing side effect that sometimes occurs with the continued use of phenytoin is gingival hyperplasia. The gums may even grow over the teeth. This most often occurs in children, rarely in adults. Frequent brushing is essential to remove food particles and prevent gingival infection. Hyperplasia may be lessened by frequent massage of the gums. Occasional application of steroid creams may help to prevent excessive overgrowth. In some patients oral surgery is required to remove excess gingiva.

Visual difficulties, motor incoordination, and a staggering gait are prominent signs of phenytoin, phenobarbital, and primidone overdose; patients should be advised to consult their physicians immediately. Because blood dyscrasias are possible, though rare, side effects of most antiepileptic medications, some physicians check their patients' white blood counts and hemoglobin levels every six months.

Consistency in taking the prescribed amount of medication is absolutely essential for the control of seizures. Taking the drug at mealtime or bedtime helps some people maintain a regular schedule, and placing the days' supply in a separate container so that any missed doses are evident is another aid. Phenytoin and phenobarbital may be taken in one daily dose, but primidone and ethosuximide are best taken in three or four daily doses.

If phenytoin must be given parenterally, the I.V. route is preferred as the drug is absorbed poorly from muscle. Intravenous phenytoin must be given slowly, no faster than 50 mg. per minute. Rapid administration may depress myocardial function and produce cardiac arrhythmias and possibly cardiac arrest. Phenytoin must be given by I.V. push. It cannot be diluted and administered in the I.V. fluid because it precipitates within minutes. Since the pH of Dilantin is near 12, it is very irritating to the veins, and the nurse should watch closely for signs of phlebitis near the I.V. site.

People with epilepsy need to be closely monitored during the dose adjustment period because individuals differ in the rate at which they metabolize drugs. Anticonvulsant levels may be elevated as a result of interaction with some drugs. Phenytoin levels have been shown to increase as a result of interaction with isoniazid, disulfiram (Antabuse), and anticoagulants, especially bishydroxycoumarin (Dicumarol)(11). Potential interactions exist between phenytoin and other medications or alcohol. Concomitant administration of phenobarbital and phenytoin may cause a decrease in phenytoin levels; withdrawal of the phenobarbital can then result in phenytoin toxicity(12). The patient should be certain that any physician who treats him is aware of the antiepileptic medications he is taking. Illnesses affecting hepatic or kidney function slow the metabolism or excretion of antiepileptic medications.

In the late 1960s, a laboratory test called gas liquid chromatography (GLC) was developed that accurately measures the concentration of drugs in the blood. This test requires at least 2 c.c. of blood and takes several hours to obtain results. The recently perfected Enzyme Multiple Immunoassay Technique (EMIT) provides information from a fingerstick blood sample about the concentration of some antiepileptic drugs. This is especially helpful in following outpatients because test results are available in minutes. These laboratory aids help physicians to adjust dosages so that the patient has an adequate amount of drug for seizure control with minimal side effects. They are especially valuable when there is a question of patient compliance with the drug therapy.

The epileptic should be aware of other events which may lower his seizure threshold. He should know that extreme emotional or physical stress may precipitate an attack. Excessive fluid retention—premenstrual edema, for example—may increase the incidence of seizures and can be treated with a mild diuretic. Alcohol may lower the seizure threshold, so excessive use of alcohol is not advisable. Most patients can safely drink an occasional cocktail.

ACUTE NURSING CARE

When planning the care for a patient hospitalized with epilepsy, the nurse must consider the type and frequency of seizure activity. The patient should be ambulatory and permitted as much freedom as possible unless he has frequent uncontrolled seizures. Many people who have auras learn to go to bed or lie on the floor and call for assistance before secondary generalization occurs. Sometimes the nurse is alerted to an ongoing seizure by the epileptic cry at the start of a generalized seizure.

When a generalized seizure occurs, the nurse stays with the patient, and assists him to lie down. If possible, a padded tongue blade or rolled wash cloth is placed between the patient's teeth to prevent tongue biting. If the teeth are already clenched, they should not be forced open because any damage to the tongue has already occurred, and further trauma may be inflicted by breaking the teeth(13).

If the patient is on the floor, his head may be protected by placing a pillow or folded blanket under it or the nurse may kneel and cradle his head on her lap, maintaining it as much as possible in hyperextension. Tight clothing around the neck and belts should be loosened to allow respiratory excursion. The patient's extremities should not be restrained because fractures may result.

The patient's head should be maintained in a lateral dependent, and hyperextended position to clear the airway. As soon as the clonic phase ceases, he should be turned to his side to promote drainage of accumulated secretions. Pharyngeal suctioning may be necessary.

Most seizures stop in four to five minutes. A seizure that stops spontaneously is not an emergency. But if a patient seems to pass from one seizure to another without regaining consciousness, he could be in status epilepticus and a physician should be notified immediately.

STATUS EPILEPTICUS

The most frequent cause of status epilepticus is failure to take the prescribed dose of antiepileptic medication.

Status epilepticus is a medical emergency that threatens the patient's life. Establishing an adequate airway is the first step in the management. Oral airway and suctioning must be instituted to protect the patient against aspiration and subsequent pulmonary involvement. In severe or protracted cases, a tracheostomy may be performed. Drug therapy is directed toward arresting the seizure activity, but the physician must also consider the cause of the seizure in his approach to the therapy.

The use of diazepam (Valium) has proved to be valuable in arresting status epilepticus. It can be injected directly into the vein or in a saline or dextrose infusion over a two-minute period. Following the diazepam, phenobarbital and phenytoin must also be given to control the seizures on a long-term basis. When all other drug and adjunctive means fail, the use of generalized anesthesia and curare may be required.

The most serious complications of status epilepticus include death or permanent brain damage from hyperpyrexia and hypoxia. In addition, the therapy necessary to control status epilepticus may in itself, cause cardiac or respiratory arrest.

Besides protecting the patient from injury during any seizure, observing him carefully is important particularly if the type of seizure disorder has not been diagnosed. Syncopal spells and hysteria may mimic seizure activity, and the observations made during a seizure often provide valuable data.

These are the most important questions to keep in mind as the nurse makes these observations:

- *Where did the seizure start and how did it progress?* If the seizure is of focal origin, these observations will help locate the underlying lesion. Convulsive movements may be minimal or absent in syncope or hysterical episodes.
- *How long did the seizure last?* Most seizures and syncopal spells last only a few minutes. Hysterical episodes tend to last longer.
- *Were there any pupil changes?* In a true generalized seizure, the pupils may be dilated and nonreactive to light. If the seizure is of focal origin, the eyes may *point away* from the irritating focus. Pupillary changes do not occur in hysterical episodes and may or may not be present during syncope.
- *Was the patient incontinent of urine or feces?* Incontinence occurs in about 50 percent of generalized seizures, particularly if the bladder is full or nearly full. Incontinence is rare during syncopal or hysterical episodes.
- *Were reflexes normal after seizure?* The Babinski reflex is checked by stroking the lateral planter surface of the foot. The normal response is plantar flexion of the large toe; the abnormal is dorsiflexion of the large toe and may be elicited after a generalized seizure but usually not after a hysterical episode.

After the patient regains consciousness, he should be asked if he experienced any unusual sensations before the seizure. His answers may add information about the location of a focal abnormality. Simple descriptive terms are the best to record what is seen, including the time sequence, and what the patient recalls. Labels should not be attached to the events observed because the different use of the various terms to describe seizures may lead to confusion rather than clarification.

LONG-TERM NURSING CARE

From the time a person is diagnosed as having epilepsy, fears and misconceptions about the disease and treatment mount. Nurses can help dispel the myths even as they empathize with the physiological, social, and emotional changes and frustrations that the patient, family, and friends encounter.

Controversy about the inheritance of epilepsy has raged for years. Due to ignorance, the marriage of epileptics formerly was prohibited in the United States and still is in some other countries. Today epilepsy is no longer a statutory bar to marriage anywhere in the United States.

Most neurologists agree that there is a heredity factor in seizure disorders, but that the kind of epilepsy, the age of onset, number of siblings or relatives affected, and other factors must be considered in the genetic counseling of an epileptic who wishes to become a parent. We cannot begin to present the multiple factors which should be considered in genetic counseling. The nurse's responsibility is to refer the concerned person to a neurologist.

Parents of an affected child frequently ask about his intelligence, ability to learn, or about limiting his activity. Will he be "different?" As with any chronic illness, there are stages in adaptation. Initially, shock and denial are accompanied by some vague belief that the epilepsy may go away, and there may be reluctance to follow the medical regimen necessary for an individual to gain "control" of his life.

Parents can be assisted during this stage to help their child. The child epileptic must not think of himself as different or have so many constraints on his activity that other children see vast differences. A regular schedule of activity, sleep, and recreation should be followed, stressful situations kept to a minimum, and activities encouraged to help the child develop physical and emotional strength.

Medication *must* be taken regularly. A common misunderstanding is that once seizures are controlled, the medication may be discontinued. Nurses may meet adolescent patients who are having seizures after some years of freedom from them. A variety of reasons could account for this: angry at being "different," the adolescent may have stopped his medication; a rapid growth rate or heightened stress at home or school may be increasing the amount of medication required for seizure control.

The activity of affected persons, as a general rule, should not be limited. Common sense should be employed in restricting athletic participation. The epileptic in good control should be able to swim or ride a bicycle with a companion, or participate in field sports, but high-risk recreations like skin-diving or mountain climbing which may endanger both the epileptic's life or another's require much consideration.

Cognitive abilities vary among people with epilepsy as they do with the general population. Epilepsy and intellectual impairment are not synonymous. The apparent mental impairment of some epileptic children may be related to an inability to achieve their greatest potential because of deficient educational and social opportunities. However, brain damage and secondary intellectual impairment can result from uncontrolled seizures that cause prolonged hypoxia. Also, if a person repeatedly falls during seizures and strikes his head, residual brain damage may occur.

In assisting a patient and his family to deal with the stigma of epilepsy, the nurse can be extremely helpful if she knows the community's resources. The Epilepsy Foundation of America in Washington, D.C., is a national organization that provides literature and information on legal aspects, the employment of epileptics, first aid treatment, and so forth.

The adolescent epileptic faces new crises as he makes decisions about driving, dating, continued education, and employment. The epileptic's opportunity, ability, and ambition at this time are as much a function of his own motivation and achievement as they are of the control of seizures. Individuals should be counselled toward the realization of their own potential.

Employment of an epileptic should be based on his interest, capabilities, and goals, as with any applicant. Few work restrictions are necessary for the employee whose seizures are controlled. Claiming that insurance rates prohibit the employment of epileptics is incorrect. There is conclusive proof that epileptic individuals doing the same job as nonepileptics have no greater number of claims(14). Accident and sickness rates are good, if not better, than rates for nonepileptic persons(15). With such statistics, it may be to an employer's advantage to hire an epileptic if his interest and skills meet the employer's need.

Many state legislatures have enacted the Second Injury Fund, an extension of the workman's compensation fund which compensates employees for disabilities resulting from the job. The Second Injury Fund is an aid to the employer of previously handicapped people because it limits the employer's liability to the amount arising from the second injury. Epileptics should inform employers of their epileptic disorder in order to collect compensation for an injury sustained during an on-the-job seizure.

Sensible preventive measures include wearing a medical-alert bracelet, available in most drug stores, and carrying a wallet card that states the facts pertinent to the epileptic condition. If necessary, the person with akinetic epilepsy should wear a football helmet to prevent brain injury from repeated falls.

Except in unusual cases, the epileptic person's diet need be no different than a normal person's. Most physicians prescribe moderation in all that the epileptic person does, whether it is eating or another activity. He should be encouraged to take part in sports, attend school to the level of his achievement, work and eat as does the general population.

REFERENCES
1. SCHMIDT, R. P., AND WILDER, B. J. *Epilepsy*. Philadelphia, F. A. Davis Co., 1958, p. 2.
2. *Ibid.*, p. 7.
3. *Ibid.*, p. 11.
4. *Ibid.*, pp. 4-5.
5. WILLIAMS, ANNE. Classification and diagnosis of epilepsy. *Nurs. Clin.NorthAm.* 9:758. Dec. 1974.
6. SCHMIDT, *op.cit.*, p. 2.
7. TEMPKIN, OWSEL. *The Falling Sickness, rev. ed.* Baltimore, Johns Hopkins University Press, 1971, p. 337.
8. BARROW, R. L., AND FABINO, H. D. *Epilepsy and the Law*. New York, Harper and Brothers, 1956, p. 5.
9. SCHMIDT, *op.cit.*, p. 170.
10. *Ibid.*, p. 174.
11. HANSTEN, P. D. *Drug Interactions. 3rd ed.* Philadelphia, Lea & Febiger, 1975, pp. 33-34, 38, 140.
12. *Ibid.*, pp. 135-136.
13. CARINI, ESTA, AND OWENS, GUY. *Neurological and Neurosurgical Nursing.* 5th ed. St. Louis, C. V. Mosby Co., 1974, p. 161.
14. *Ibid.*, p. 157.
15. LIONE, J. G. Convulsive disorders in a working population. *J.Occup.Med.* 3:369-373. Aug. 1961.

Bringing Epilepsy Out of the Closet

LAURALE HARKNESS

The name "epilepsy" can create more handicaps than the disorder itself, says this nurse who started a campus group to battle stigma and discrimination.

Most nurses can recall at least one lecture on epilepsy in their basic nursing program. All too often the physiological aspects are overemphasized and the psychosocial aspects neglected. Epilepsy is the only common physical disorder whose name frequently creates more handicaps than the disturbance itself(1).

Epilepsy has a history similar to that of mental illness. Thinking that evil spirits dwelt in the person, men employed techniques like trephining to let them out. In the Bible a man begs Jesus to remove the evil spirit from his son's body! "A spirit taketh him, and he suddenly crieth out; and it teareth him that he foameth. . . ."(2). This evil-spirit concept has persisted into present times.

The author of a nurses' textbook of 1898 states that insanity is connected with other nervous diseases; he names several, including an "epileptic insanity"(3). The bizarre behavior accompanying an epileptic seizure is often likened to that of a schizophrenic or manic-depressive individual. In our culture, there is a tendency to categorize epileptics as being out of control, a most degrading and shameful classification.

For a working definition, I refer to epilepsy as a disorder of nerve cell function in the brain characterized by episodes of impaired consciousness that may or may not be associated with convulsions(4). In many

---

MS. HARKNESS *received her B.S.N. from the University of Wisconsin-Eau Claire School of Nursing last June and began working as a staff nurse at University Hospital, Minneapolis, Minn. While a senior student, she started the campus group for epileptics which she describes in this article.*

cases, the cause is unknown. Although electroencephalography is a useful diagnostic tool, the incidence of normal EEGs among people who have seizures "is exceedingly high"(5). An estimated 2 percent of the population of the United States, or 4 million people, suffer from this disorder(6).

Ninety percent of all epileptics have their first seizures before the age of 20. Initial symptoms are commonly noticed in one of three periods: the first two years of life, ages five to seven years, and the onset of puberty(7). During this last period, the peer group becomes increasingly important. Conformity to its norms is essential for the development of a positive body image.

The epileptic child is frequently ridiculed by his classmates for his strange behavior. A negative body image results and is extremely difficult to correct, even though 90 percent of epileptics function normally in society(8). Unfortunately, this is usually possible only through deception. The epileptic simply lies about his disorder. Why is this necessary?

Generally, people express compassion toward the sick and disabled. The person with epilepsy, however, has been viewed as sinister and criminal(9).

Negative attitudes toward epilepsy are deep-rooted and are reflected in many ways. The Epilepsy Foundation reported a survey done by McDaniel(10). People who hire applicants for business or schools were asked to rank the desirability of employees with various kinds of disabilities. Epilepsy was ranked thirteenth, with personal directors and school administrators giving preference to amputees, the blind, the deaf, and many others. Because a controlled epileptic has a work potential equal to that of any healthy adult, it is easy to see that a lack of understanding promotes depression and defensiveness in epileptics.

The laws pertaining to epileptics further complicate their situation(11). As recently as 1960, seven states still applied antimarriage laws to epileptics. By 1969, only West Virginia had such laws. In 13 states, in 1960, institutionalized epileptics were subject to sterilization and, in six other states, a board decided whether an epileptic was to undergo sterilization(12). Fortunately, eugenic sterilization laws in the United States have been virtually abandoned in the past decade(11). There were anti-immigration laws against epileptics in the United States until 1968, and several states in 1972 still forbade their driving under any circumstances(13).

START OF A CAMPUS PROJECT

In view of the social attitudes, employment discrimination, and legal restraints, I undertook a campuswide project to support students with epilepsy and marshall resources to educate the public. As a senior nursing student and an epileptic, I have a keen interest in the disorder. My condition has been completely controlled for four-and-one-half years. I began having seizures at the age of 12 and was diagnosed and completely controlled by 18. I've led a relatively normal life—swimming, dancing, going to proms, and attending a school of nursing. My concern over the treatment of epileptics stems from the Navy Nurse Corps' rejection of my application because of my disorder. This was an extremely traumatic experience and brought into sharp focus the bias that exists toward me and others with epilepsy.

To search out other epileptics on campus was my hardest task. Most epileptics choose to remain anonymous because of past rejection or fear of future rejection. An organizational meeting was announced by posters and the campus newspaper.

The first student arrived about five minutes late and stood outside the door for a couple of minutes before he ventured in. He fidgeted with his clothes, looked anxious and very awkward. This behavior manifested the difficulty an epileptic has in admitting his disorder to strangers, especially as physicians, parents, and teachers have instructed him to conceal it. He then paced in and out, continuing to show apprehension.

Eight persons came. Most, for the first time in their lives, found other epileptics who shared their discouragement. They talked about their personal experiences. Frequently expressed comments were "It feels so good to talk with others like myself" and "An epileptic has to lead a normal life."

AN IDEA SESSION

The second meeting, two weeks later, was an idea session. We determined to establish the group as an official university organization; it is now known as the Eau Claire Epilepsy Collective (ECEC). Membership has stabilized at 10. Two of us are community members, the rest are students.

The purposes are to support members and provide public education. Besides mutual sharing, support includes encouraging epileptics to follow their medical regimens, use Medic Alert bracelets, and take part in cultural and social activities other than drinking, as alcohol stimulates seizures. Also, the group decided to help students buy medication at a discount through the National Epilepsy League.

At this second session, we prepared a fact sheet about epilepsy and organized to approach department chairmen about meeting their faculties. Group representatives have now discussed their experiences and the purpose of ECEC with an estimated 400 faculty members. They have offered us every opportunity to teach our classmates and to address special education classes and present and future elementary school teachers. Articles have been featured in the campus and local papers.

At the close of the academic year, ECEC extended its activities for 1973-1974, including the possible establishment of groups in local high schools. A distinguished neurologist will speak on epilepsy, without charge, to interested groups.

The social stigma remains, but ECEC's acceptance from the university faculty tells us that the barrier is coming down on this campus. The public is beginning to listen, even to assist us in alleviating discrimination.

REFERENCES

1. LIVINGSTON, SAMUEL. *Living with Epileptic Seizures.* Springfield, Ill., Charles C Thomas, Publisher, 1963, p. 211.
2. LUKE 9:39.
3. WISE, P. M. *A Textbook for Training Schools for Nurses.* New York, G. P. Putnam's Sons, 1898, vol. 2, p. 136.
4. LIVINGSTON, *op.cit.,* p. 3.
5. LIVINGSTON, SAMUEL. *Comprehensive Management of Epilepsy in Infancy, Childhood and Adolescence.* Springfield, Ill., Charles C Thomas, Publisher, 1972, pp. 10-11.
6. Organized effort continues to help the epileptic. *Horizon* (National Epilepsy League, Chicago) Fall 1972, p. 1.
7. LIVINGSTON, SAMUEL. *Comprehensive Management of Epilepsy in Infancy, Childhood and Adolescence.* Springfield, Ill., Charles C Thomas. Publisher, 1972, *op.cit.,* p. 6.
8. SANDS, HARRY, AND SEAVER, JACQUELINE. *Epilepsy: Today's Encouraging Outlook.* (Public Affairs Pamphlet No. 387) New York, Public Affairs Committee, 1966.
9. KEMP, ROBERT. *Understanding Epilepsy.* London, Tavistock Publications, 1963, pp. 49-50.
10. RATING educational need; rejection. *National Spokesman* (Epilepsy Foundation of America) 5:1, June 1972.
11. LIVINGSTON, SAMUEL. *Comprehensive Management of Epilepsy in Infancy, Childhood and Adolescence.* Springfield, Ill., Charles C Thomas, Publisher, 1972, *op.cit.,* pp. 533-543.
12. LENNOX, W. G. *Epilepsy and Related Disorders.* Boston, Mass., Little, Brown and Co., vol. 2, 1960, p. 985.
13. BOSHES, L. D., AND GIBBS, F. A. *Epilepsy Handbook.* 2d ed. Springfield, Ill., Charles C Thomas, Publisher, 1972, p. 156.

Levodopa and Parkinsonism

MARILYN BEATON ROBINSON

> *Since 1968, more than 150 individuals with parkinsonism have been treated with levodopa at the Burke Rehabilitation Center. This author discusses parkinsonism, levodopa therapy, and the nursing techniques used in rehabilitating these patients.*

It is satisfying and rewarding to see a patient with parkinsonism achieve some independence and again contribute to his family and community. Only a few years ago, he would have been admitted to a chronic care facility with no hope of improvement.

Parkinsonism is a fairly common, disabling, movement disorder caused by dysfunction of the extrapyramidal system. There are 90 to 110 cases per 100,000 people and an annual incidence of 20 cases per 100,000 people in the United States(1). Parkinsonism shortens life, and many patients develop various degrees of disability within four to five years. The longer the disease continues, the more disabling it becomes, with consequent loss of independence.

Effective treatment for parkinsonism has been sought for over a century. Nearly fifty years after James Parkinson described this entity in 1871, the anticholinergic drugs were discovered to mitigate some of its symptoms. They only partially relieved tremor and rigidity, however, and did not influence the progress of the disease. Thalamic surgery sometimes suppressed symptoms on the contralateral side, but effects were unpredictable, occasionally lasting only a few months.

L-3,4-dihydroxyphenylaine (levodopa) was first isolated in 1913, but

---

MS. ROBINSON *(Westchester School of Nursing, Valhalla, N.Y.) is the charge nurse in the Parkinson's disease outpatient clinic at Burke Rehabilitation Center, White Plains, N.Y. She is also research assistant for the Parkinson's disease project being conducted at the center.*

it was not until 1960 that dopamine, its metabolite, was found to be deficient in the brains of patients with parkinsonism. Although dopamine does not readily enter the brain, it was predicted that levodopa would elevate brain dopamine levels. Clinical trials of oral levodopa in the 1960's demonstrated dramatic relief of symptoms in most cases. At the present time, levodopa is the therapy of choice for parkinsonism.

Initially the patient may complain of vague muscular pain and weakness or numbness of an extremity. The onset is insidious and so mild that it sometimes attributed to other conditions, such as fatigue, anxiety, or "rheumatism." Mild tremor in an extremity is often the first symptom, followed by rigidity and difficulty initiating movement (akinesia). Slowness of movement (bradykinesia) may appear simultaneously. Occasionally, rigidity is the prevailing symptom, with no sign of tremor. As the disease progresses, rhythmical interruption of passive range of motion (cogwheel rigidity) may occur in one or more extremities.

Mild resistive (plastic) or almost totally resistive (lead pipe) rigidity may develop as well as diminished voice volume and facial expression (mask facies), drooling (sialorrhea), oily, shiny skin with desquamation at the hair line (seborrhea), abnormally small handwriting trailing off at an angle (micographia), spasm of the eyelids (blephorospasm), small mincing steps with increasingly rapid propulsive or retropulsive pace (festination), voluntary motion slowing to a complete stop (freezing), inability to catch oneself after losing balance (loss of righting reflexes), mild flexion of the joints (simian posture), and difficulty swallowing (dysphagia). These symptoms are progressive and usually lead to severe disability.

Parkinsonism may be idiopathic, post-encephalitic, or drug-induced. Some features of parkinsonism can result from manganese dust or carbon monoxide inhalation as well as from toxic doses of reserpine or the phenothiazines.

METHODS OF EVALUATION

There are several qualitative rating scales to evaluate the extent of the disease. The one developed by Margaret Hoehn and Melvin Yahr is used by clinicians most frequently.

STAGE I: Unilateral involvement only.
STAGE II: Bilateral involvement only.
STAGE III: Impaired postural and righting reflexes. Disability mild to moderate.
STAGE IV: Fully developed, severe disease. Disability marked.
STAGE V: Confinement to bed or wheelchair(2).

A simple, quantitative method of evaluation, the Motility Index, has been developed at Burke Rehabilitation Center. The MI enables us to assign patients to the above stages and to follow the patient's progress objectively while he is receiving chronic levodopa therapy(3-5).

One of the most consistent pathological abnormalities of parkinsonism is damage to or loss of melanin-containing cells in the compact layer of the substantia nigra of the midbrain. These cells send axons to the corpus striatum (caudate nucleus and putamen), and their synaptic endings in the striatum are rich in dopamine(6). Patients suffering with parkinsonism have decreased concentrations of dopamine in the striatum and substantia nigra(7). Reasoning that dopamine loss might account for the movement disorders of parkinsonism, investigators tried to replenish dopamine levels(8-10). Dopamine, an aromatic amino acid, does not cross the blood-brain barrier, and, therefore, has no effect on parkinsonism. However, levodopa, the immediate metabolic precursor of dopamine, does cross the barrier and is readily decarboxylated to dopamine in brain tissue and ameliorates the symptoms of parkinsonism.

Levodopa is administered in tablets or capsule form. The 0.5 Gm. tablet is scored and easily halved. The initial dosage is 0.5 Gm. This is increased in small increments to avoid untoward effects such as nausea and postural hypotension. Some patients can tolerate a dose increase as great as 0.5 Gm. daily until 1.5 Gms. are reached, and then 0.5 Gm. every second day until approximately 3.0 Gms. have been reached. However, others require dose increments as low as 100 mg. every few days. There is no standard maximum optimal dose of levodopa, and reaching the proper maintenance doses for each patient is a matter of clinical judgment. In general, the dose should be increased until maximal response is achieved and continues, or until side effects occur. Reduction of the daily dose by 0.5 Gm. to 1.0 Gm. usually abolishes toxic effects. Levodopa is then continued at the lower dose in chronic treatment with some variation of dose upward or downward as side effects or suboptimal response dictate. Hospitalization during the initial dose adjustment is unnecessary unless the patient is debilitated or is in stage IV or V.

Levodopa should never be taken on an empty stomach, because of its emetic property. Our patients commonly experience gastrointestinal disturbances, especially during the initial phase of treatment. Nausea, with occasional vomiting and anorexia, may persist for several weeks, but can be controlled with antacids taken before meals, by taking the levodopa during or immediately after meals, or with a half glass of milk prior to between-meal medication. If this regimen is followed routinely, these unpleasant side effects eventually subside.

The response to levodopa is gradual and variable. During the first two weeks, the patient's motility may decline and his condition actually worsen. There is no reasonable explanation for this mild exacerbation of symptoms. Ordinarily, the patient reports a subtle feeling of well-being. He will notice a gradual reduction of rigidity and associated symptoms with maximal and sustained response to the medication. Patients who respond well to levodopa usually improve by a full stage after three to six months of therapy. Some of our patients who were in stage I or II became virtually symptom free within a year although mild tremor reappears during stressful situations. Micrographia, voice volume and articulation, simian posture, and loss of reflex arm swing improve dramatically. Tremor and loss of righting reflexes are the last symptoms to disappear. If levodopa is withdrawn, the symptoms usually reappear within three or four days, but in reverse order.

An "on-off" effect has been described by several of our patients after approximately two years of therapy. They may have progressed from stage IV to stage II, but several times during the day they suddenly become rigid, tremulous, and akinetic. While "on," they are mobile, but experience dyskinesia. The mechanism behind this phenomenon is unknown. By splitting the daily dose into one-hour or two-hour intervals, we are able to partially control this variance. Patients probably will require levodopa therapy and periodic evaluation for the rest of their lives.

ADJUNCTIVE DRUGS

The anticholinergic drugs have helped alleviate the rigidity, temor, and sialorrhea of parkinsonism. They are continued, in most instances, during levodopa therapy. It appears that they synergistically enhance the actions of levodopa.

The side effects of anticholinergic drugs can be confused with the toxic effects of levodopa. Ordinarily, the anticholinergic dosage is decreased to minimal levels after the initiation of levodopa therapy. Some anticholinergics have a cumulative effect. Many patients tolerate small doses for several years, and then develop hypersensitivity. Dryness of the mouth, followed by dilated pupils and blurred vision, may be the only indication of toxicity, but irritability, restlessness, confusion, disorientation, and visual hallucinations may occur. Reduction of the dose or total withdrawal may be necessary.

The antihistamine diphenhydramine hydrochloride (Benadryl) has mild antiparkinsonism as well as sedative properties. It is often prescribed in conjunction with one of the synthetic anticholinergics, and can be taken at bedtime to induce relaxation and sleep.

There are drugs which cause pseudoparkinsonism, are antagonistic to levodopa, or can be used as an antidote to levodopa-induced toxicity. Rauwolfia alkaloids, such as reserpine, cause pseudoparkinsonism by depleting the store of biogenic amines in the brain, including dopamine. The phenothiazine derivatives also cause parkinsonism, perhaps by blocking striatal dopamine receptors. This condition resembles reserpine-induced dopamine deficiency. Pyridoxine (vitamin B_6), a co-factor of the enzyme dopa-decarboxylase, reverses the therapeutic effect of levodopa, probably by enhancing the decarboxylation of levodopa outside the brain, thereby decreasing the availability of dopamine to the striatum. Pyridoxine has been used occasionally in small doses (5-7.5 mg.) to relieve the side effects of levodopa and allow therapy to continue uninterrupted. A multivitamin, Larobec, does not contain pyridoxine and is now available for levodopa-treated patients.

Monoamine oxidase (MAO) inhibitors are strongly contraindicated because they block the metabolism of dopamine and produce a dangerous hypertensive response in combination with levodopa. Barbiturates may produce paradoxical excitement in the elderly patient. For the same reason, hypnotic drugs should be avoided whenever possible. Diazepam (Valium) 2-5 mg. or Benadryl 25-50 mg. are preferred if a sedative is required.

Chronic self-medication by the elderly patient is one of the greatest challenges to the clinical nurse. A patient may decide to take a multivitamin other than Larobec. Many patients do not regard vitamin preparations or over-the-counter remedies as drugs. A patient may decide to substitute or omit certain medications. Also, a physician who is unfamiliar with the patient may prescribe drugs which may be contraindicated with levodopa therapy. The nurse should be aware of every medication the patient is taking, their composition, and the amounts taken daily.

Forgetfulness and confusion cause many dosage errors. The spouse or a responsible family member should be instructed in administering the daily medications and be provided with a written list which includes the names, amounts, and time when they must be taken. A pill box should be used and the day's medications placed in it each morning. This eliminates the constant use of the stock bottles and ensures at least that a forgetful patient does not exceed his daily requirements. Patients who are capable of self-medication should also be given a list with precise instructions. It is imperative that they understand that they must not alter the dosage of levodopa or discontinue their anticholinergic drug without first consulting the prescribing physician.

The patient may be taking several adjunctive and concomitant drugs. Dosage errors will be reduced if all medication bottles are clearly labeled. Availability of the nurse on the telephone can help to untangle misunderstandings and confusion. Our patients know they can call at any time during the day if they have questions or problems. However, there is no guarantee, despite constant follow-up, that the patient responsible for his own medications will take them accurately. This must be considered in evaluating a patient's response to treatment.

MANAGING LEVODOPA SIDE EFFECTS

The side effects encountered most often by our patients are the dyskinesias, or abnormal involuntary movements. These usually occur during periods of greatest motility and include grimacing, lip smacking, tongue clicking and protrusion, squinting, head bobbing, extension-flexion and rotation of the neck and shoulder, abnormal movements of the intercostal muscles and diaphragm that cause bizarre breathing patterns, and abnormal rotation of an extremity, usually the forelimb, hand, or foot. These may occur at dosages of less than 2.0 Gms. The onset can be insidious or abrupt. They often occur at the same time each day, for instance, 30 minutes after taking the noon dose. Spreading the medication, as with the "on-off" effect, may alleviate mild dyskinesia.

The majority of patients have hypotension before and during therapy. The systolic pressure can fall to 100 mm. Hg or lower. Patients do not seem to be affected by this phenomenon, but it is important to establish a base norm before therapy begins. Orthostatic hypotension, defined as a drop in systolic pressure of 30 mm. Hg between supine and standing pressures, or a drop to below 100 mm. Hg, may or may not cause symptoms. Episodes of vertigo, light-headedness, and syncopal attacks can occur.

Levodopa-related mental confusion, disorientation, and hallucinations must not be confused with the similar toxic effects of other drugs, particularly the anticholinergics. If the aberrant behavior appears abruptly after titration to maximal levodopa dosage, an immediate reduction or complete withdrawal is indicated. Gradual retitration to a lower dose after the symptoms clear can then be initiated. A preexisting severe organic dementia may be exposed as the patient's parkinsonism improves. This is unfortunate because the therapeutic response may be negated by the more dominant symptoms of dementia and a once docile, cooperative patient will then present a difficult care problem.

Insomnia and restlessness are sometimes reported. An understanding of the patient's sleep habits should be elicited from relatives. The patient may be fearful of the night, particularly in a hospital environment, present mild organic dementia, or drug sensitivity. Encouraging him to retire later than usual and holding his last dose of levodopa and a sedative until the later hour may be the only remedy necessary.

Parkinsonism usually occurs among patients in the age group with a high incidence of cardiovascular disease, which is the leading cause of death among the United States population as a whole, as well as among those afflicted with parkinsonism(2). Evidence of cardiovascular problems frequently appears on the pretreatment electrocardiogram, and may continue throughout therapy. If tachycardia or palpitations appear abruptly with no previously recorded episodes, levodopa should be discontinued to determine whether it is the causative factor. If the symptoms subside, the levodopa can be retitrated slowly to a lower maximal dose, or to the previous dose if it is established that the arrhythmia was not due to levodopa toxicity.

Flushing, accompanied by hot flashes, has been described by four of our patients. This may occur once or twice at the same time each day and will diminish in intensity and disappear gradually after the dosage has been reduced.

An occasional patient voids pink or bright red urine which turns black when exposed to air. This is caused by the metabolites of dopamine. A female patient may have post-menopausal spotting. This may be related to dopamine stimulation of hypothalamic hormone releasing factors, but a primary urinary tract infection or gynecological abnormality must be ruled out. Salty, metallic, or "unusual" taste sensations have been reported. Foul body odor can be attributed to the metabolites of levodopa. Patients should be informed of these side effects because they can cause considerable anxiety. Surprisingly, the dyskinesias, with the exception of bizarre breathing, may not worry patients to any great degree, probably because they are used to the abnormal tremulous movements associated with parkinsonism.

NURSING MANAGEMENT

The patient's weight should be recorded once a week while he is hospitalized, and during each out-patient visit. Because levodopa has diuretic properties, there may be an initial weight loss and this may be compounded by anorexia and nausea(11). Asking relatives to describe the patient's nutritional habits can help in determining the need for supplemental high caloric foods. Multiple, small, attractive meals encourage higher caloric intake. Food should be arranged so that the patient can eat as independently as possible. A patient in stage III to V may have to eat foods like peas and corn with a spoon. Meat should be cut before it is presented to the patient. It is tempting to offer a semi-soft diet so meals are eaten quickly, but a regular diet should be continued unless dysphagia is present. A bib should not be used unless absolutely necessary and only during meals because this emphasizes the patient's inability to cope and embarrasses him. The Parkinson's patient needs considerably more time than usual for eating. Weight loss can result from rushing a tremulous, akinetic person through meals.

Obesity adds to the problems of the patient in stage III to V. Loss of righting reflexes occurs, and the entire spectrum of symptoms becomes pronounced. Patients in these stages lead sedentary lives, and food may compensate. A low-calorie diet and persistent counseling can foster weight loss. Motivation to lose weight can be achieved with the prospect of regained motor function as therapy continues.

Blood pressure should be taken, twice daily, sitting and standing, with at least 30 seconds between measurements if the person is hospitalized, and at each outpatient visit. Ask the patient if he experiences dizziness. If so, he may need to sit for a short while before getting out of bed, and pause after standing and before beginning to walk. Rapid postural changes may cause fleeting vertigo, loss of balance, and a fall. Since the majority of our patients are elderly and suffer from degenerative bone disease, fractures can occur and diminish or halt the rate of improvement. Fractures are also more likely to occur as levodopa permits more activity.

Fluid intake should be monitored carefully, especially if the patient is in advanced parkinsonism. Infections of the urinary tract are common. Urinary stasis is a contributing factor and results from lack of movement and insufficient fluid intake. Fluids should be offered frequently. Tremor may make drinking from a cup extremely difficult, but the patient usually can manage with flexible drinking straws.

Levodopa may cause polyuria. Urinary frequency, common in most elderly patients as a result of poor muscle tone of the bladder and sphincters, is intensified by diuresis. The patient should void as soon as he feels the urge. An overwhelming urgency may cause him unnecessary embarrassment. Nocturia, with accidental enuresis, does not necessarily indicate incontinence. Probably the patient could not get out of bed rapidly enough or the urinal was out of reach. A urinal or commode should be readily available to patients who are bradykinetic. A bathroom night light will decrease the incidence of falls experienced by ambulatory patients.

Sluggish peristalsis, due to lack of physical activity, poor muscle tone, the effect of anticholinergic drugs, and possibly the disease process itself, may cause chronic constipation. This is one of the most persistent complaints expressed by our patients. Mild laxatives should be used, such as Peri-Colace 100 mg. twice daily, or a Dulcolax 10 mg. suppository every other day. Peri-Colace is a stool softener; Dulcolax stimulates sensory nerve endings to increase peristaltic contractions. The patient should never let more than three days go by without proper elimination. Fecal impactions are not uncommon, particularly if the patient lives alone, and have occasionally necessitated hospitalization. A few of our patients have diarrhea. This is usually due to constipation, since an incomplete impaction allows fluids to seep around the fecal material and cause overflow diarrhea. A rectal examination should be done before administering an antidiarrhetic.

Bronchopneumonia is the second most frequent cause of death in patients afflicted with advanced parkinsonism(1). Rigidity and akinesia prevent moving in bed. Even if the patient can turn, he expends so much energy that he becomes exhausted and frustrated and prefers to lie in the same position indefinitely. His position should be changed every two hours during the night. Ordinary pillows, quarter-size pillows, and folded towels will protect bony prominences and maintain position. A sheepskin beneath the buttocks and heels prevents skin breakdown, and bed cradles relieve pressure and hinder contraction of the Achilles tendons. It is wise to use a loose restraint and supportive pillows while the patient is in a wheelchair since he may lean to his less involved side. Foam rubber padding in the chair seat helps prevent skin deterioration. Pressure sores are a constant threat and may lead to many weeks of rehabilitative effort.

A thorough daily bath is vitally important. Profuse perspiration from tremor and exertion, seborrhea, sialorrhea, and difficulty handling food and liquids necessitates particular attention to skin care. Oral hygiene should be given at least twice daily. Buccal tremor with consequent grinding of teeth, oral respiration, and anticholinergic drugs can cause an excessively dry mouth.

Hand rails should be installed next to the toilet and in the bathtub if the patient is in stage III to V. A chair in the shower stall or bathtub facilitates bathing. The patient will need assistance in sitting, rising, bathing his lower extremities, grooming, and dressing. Bras can be provided with front fastenings, or may be fastened in the front and turned. Velcro is very useful as a substitute for buttons and zippers when stitched to either side of openings. Rubberized shoe strings save considerable time. Loose fitting, comfortable garments should be provided. Women who wear constricting garters should be encouraged to use ordinary hose. Antiembolic stockings should be worn if dependent edema or hypotension persist.

Physical exercise is an essential adjunct to levodopa therapy. Exercise prevents contractures, stimulates circulation, prevents dependent edema, and promotes well-being. Knee- and ankle-flexion contractures are a menace and hinder levodopa response. We have had to refer several patients for orthopedic surgery before they could begin to walk. If a patient is living at home, relatives should be instructed in assisting him to ambulate. Reinforcement of exercise is absolutely necessary, or the scheduled exercise is a waste of time. If he can, the patient should reinforce his own regimen by using a stationary bicycle and by performing active resistive exercises with pulleys and weights.

A patient may respond so favorably to levodopa that he virtually has to be taught to walk again. Falling may result from over-enthusiasm and lack of skill or caution, as well as from the poor postural reflexes inherent in parkinsonism. He should be instructed to relax and to initiate ambulation slowly, and emphasis given to correct posture and automatic arm swing. Shuffling and dragging the feet are typical manifestations of parkinsonism and can become habits which are difficult to break even after a maximal response has been attained. The patient may need a reminder to lift his feet so that they clear the floor, and to take longer steps. The goal is always safer, smoother, more normal gait.

Pivotal turning is used by patients who have progressed to stage III parkinsonism and who are unable to turn easily because of irregular, festinating steps. This can cause balance loss, and is responsible for many falls. The patient can be instructed to raise his toes as he turns. This places his weight on his heels and eases the turn. Walking a large semicircle can be accomplished with longer steps and unbroken rhythm. Marching to music, walking a straight line with contact guarding, and games of catch with bean bags or handballs will reinforce his balance reflex and, combined with levodopa therapy, improve his motor function.

PSYCHOSOCIAL ASPECTS

Confirmation of the diagnosis of parkinsonism can be a severe shock to patients and their families. The public has a vague idea of the grossly debilitating effects of advanced Parkinson's disease and knows there was no hope of arresting its downhill course until the advent of levodopa. The untreated patient may have suffered for several years. The resultant anguish and depression exert a tremendous influence on the structure and quality of his family relationships. The stigma of parkinsonism is only too real to those afflicted with it and to those who live near them.

An awareness of the many problems the patient faces helps relieve friction and enables his family to support his progress.

The family should be fully acquainted with the symptoms of parkinsonism. Mask facies prevent the patient from registering emotion, and can be irritating and perplexing. A formerly gregarious, extroverted person becomes solemn, irritable, and demanding. This is sometimes translated by the family as "feeling sorry for himself." The spouse may suspect malingering, particularly if the patient experiences the dramatic "on-off" effect, caring for himself one moment and totally dependent the next. This also exasperates the medical team if they are unaware of the nature of the phenomenon. Relatives must adjust so that the patient can continue his daily schedule without feeling rushed. They should understand that he needs more time than usual for simple tasks.

The progressing symptoms force the patient to slacken pace and, as a consequence, employment may be terminated prematurely. The coordinated movements and quick reflexes needed to drive a car may be so impaired that he must stop driving. Micrographia makes it increasingly difficult to sign checks, correspond, and manage his own affairs. All this has a tremendous psychological impact on a previously dynamic person.

Unable to perform the activities of daily living, insecure while walking, embarrassed by his tremor, drooling, and blank expression, he may withdraw to the confines of home and a sedentary life. This isolates him from society and contributes to his physical problems. Reclusive habits become established, and family members sometimes adapt only too well and insist on continuing to manage the patient and his affairs.

The patient may grow to enjoy a dependent role, and not wish the situation to change. He cannot avoid the fact, however, that during treatment with levodopa he is becoming increasingly independent. Nor can his relatives, who may be more than willing to surrender their responsibilities. On the other hand, a wife may feel needed once more, her husband becoming a child replacement, and it can be most difficult to convince her that she may impede his progress by encouraging his continuing dependence on her. Satisfying his every need discourages him from discovering his evolving capabilities in response to levodopa therapy.

It is important to scrutinize the total human being when dealing with people afflicted with parkinsonism. One can readily see, even at a distance, the tremor and lack of facial expression, but the ability to communicate, his range of motion, and physical integrity, which healthy people take for granted, also may be partially or severely impaired. Parkinsonism is a degrading disease. The very fact that it is insidious and progressive dismays and depresses the patient. It is the nurse's responsibility to work with the emotional as well as physical problems generated by the disease, and to deal with his family's attitudes and their understanding of parkinsonism.

In summary, levodopa is an impressive therapeutic tool in the symptomatic relief of parkinsonism. The side effects caused by drug toxicity do not create insurmountable problems in control. Levodopa is an extremely safe drug if it is used with a thorough knowledge of the technique of administration and the ability to recognize side effects when they occur. The patient's levodopa dosage, and his adjunctive and concomitant medications must be carefully monitored.

The nurse is the liaison between the physician, patient, and his family. This is a role that can make a great difference in the quality of the patient's response to levodopa therapy.

REFERENCES

1. McDowell, F. H. The diagnosis of parkinsonism or parkinson syndrome. In *Recent Advances in Parkinson's Disease,* ed. by F. H. McDowell and C. J. Markham. Philadelphia, F. A. Davis Co., 1971, pp. 164-165.
2. Hoehn, M. M., and Yahr, M. Parkinsonism: onset, progression, and mortality. *Neurology* 17:427-442, May 1967.
3. Stern, P. H., and others. Quantitative testing of motility defects in patients after stroke. *Arch.Phys.Med.* 50:320-325. June 1969.
4. ———. Levodopa and physical therapy in treatment of patients with Parkinson's disease. *Arch.Phy.Med.* 51:273-277, May 1970.
5. ———. Levodopa effects on natural history of Parkinsonism. *Arch.Neurol.* 27:481-485, 1972.
6. Carlsson, A. Basic concepts underlying recent developments in the field of Parkinson's disease. IN *Recent Advances in Parkinson's Disease,* ed. by F. H. McDowell and C. J. Markham. Philadelphia, F. A. Davis Co., 1971, pp. 1-31
7. Hornykiewicz, O. Neurochemical pathology and pharmacology of brain dopamine and acetylcholine: Rational basis for the current drug treatment of Parkinsonism. IN *Recent Advances in Parkinson's Disease,* ed. by F. H. McDowell and C. J. Markham. Philadelphia, F. A. Davis Co., 1971, pp. 33-65.
8. Birkmayer, W., and Hornykiewicz, O. Des L-3, 4 dioxyphenylalanin (=DOPA)= Effekt bie des Parkinson Akinese. *Wien Klin.Wochenschr.* 73:787-788, Nov. 10, 1961.
9. Barbeau, A., and others. Les catecholomaines dans La Madadie de Parkinson. IN *Proceedings.* Symposium Bel-Air: Monoamines and the nervous system, held at Geneva, Sept. 1, 1961, ed. by J. de Ajuriaguerra. Geneva, Masson and Cie, 1962, p. 247.
10. Cotzias, G. C., and others. Modification of Parkinsonism—chronic treatment with L-dopa. *N.Engl.J.Med.* 280:337-345, Feb. 13, 1969.
11. Finlay, G. D., and others. Augmentation of sodium and potassium excretion, glomerular filtration rate and renal plasma flow by levodopa. *N.Engl.J.Med.* 284:865-870, Apr. 22, 1971.

From the *American Journal of Nursing* 73:1910-1911, Nov. 1973. Copyright © 1973. AJN Co.

Improving Speech in Parkinson's Disease

ELIZABETH ERB

Speech therapy classes enhanced the socialization activities of a small group of patients with Parkinson's disease.

The retired college professor and author of several books is still keen of mind but frustrated every time he wants to get an idea across in words. Little wonder that he's cantankerous at times! The governess-school teacher, mentally alert but slightly deaf, is troubled by not being able to speak clearly. The elderly junior high school teacher speaks in such low tones he can hardly be understood. His intellect unaffected, he knows what is going on around him and listens to the news telecast each evening, yet he sits silently in his chair all day long, except to call a nurse to reposition him.

These three people all have difficulty speaking due to Parkinson's disaase. We decided to start a speech class at our retirement home to give them whatever help we could. We began slowly and later adapted a few exercises we had learned from a speech therapist in the local schools. A physiotherapist helped us set up our program and continues to check on it.

Since breath control is very important in speaking, the therapy period begins with breathing exercises. The arms are raised straight above the shoulders while air is inhaled through the nose. Then the arms are lowered as air is exhaled through the mouth with a hissing sound. The hiss-

---

MS. ERB (*Reading Hospital School of Nursing, Reading, Pa.; B.A., Eastern Mennonite College, Harrisonburg, Va.; M.S., Francis Payne Bolton School of Nursing, Western Reserve University, Cleveland, Ohio*) *was a missionary nurse in India for 25 years. She retired in 1971 because of advanced Parkinsonism, and has been teaching the speech therapy class described in this article.*

ing makes patients aware of the amount of air being exhaled, and they are encouraged to lengthen the hissing time.

In another breathing exercise, the arms are extended forward from the body at a 90° angle and then returned to a resting position. Or the arms may be extended directly outward from the shoulders horizontally, and a flying action simulated to give range of motion to the shoulder. Of these three exercises, the upward arm extension seems to work best for breath control. A different technique is to have the patient take a deep breath and count out loud as long as possible, using only the exhaled air of that one breath. He is encouraged to increase the number of digits he can count loudly.

Breathing exercises are exhausting and should not be carried out too long, especially if the patient is severely handicapped. Tongue, jaw, and lip exercises provide a relaxing change. Each patient is given a hand mirror so that he may see his own progress. First, the tongue is extended from the mouth. The tip of the tongue is then moved upward toward the nose as far as possible, then downward toward the chin as far as possible. After this, the tongue is curled over the lips, and in this curled position is moved from side to side, first over the upper lip and then over the lower, as though removing food particles from the lips. After drawing his tongue back and while keeping his mouth closed, the patient moves the tip of his tongue freely up and down behind his teeth. Five repetitions of each exercise are adequate for one class period, provided the patient practices outside of class periods.

After these initial exercises, we practice saying the syllable "lah." The tongue is set against the inner surface of the upper front teeth, then drawn backwards, and dropped to the floor of the mouth as the mouth is opened fully.

Jaw exercises are simple opening and closing, saying "ah" when opening the jaw and "e" when closing it. The jaw exercises facilitate a purposeful opening of the mouth, relaxing the muscles of the jaw and of the throat so that the air passages will be open for breathing and speaking. Because Parkinsonian patients tend to keep their mouths open almost constantly, special emphasis must be given to closing the jaws completely when saying "e." We also practice saying "oo-ee," pursing the lips to say "oo" and stretching them into a big smile to say "ee," to loosen the lip muscles.

Drills follow the exercises. One of the simplest drills is to list words using the "oo" and "ee" sounds—open, over, clover, evening, free, beam—and then pronounce each word clearly at least five times.

Another technique for improving pronunciation is to go through the alphabet and pick out those letters which are hampering understandable speech. Phonetic sentences and phrases can be constructed to be read aloud for practice:

Do ducks dive in deep water?
This thread is twisted and tangled.
Little lambs leap with delight on the green lawn.
The west winds were whispering in the weeping willow trees.

One member of our class is particularly apt to speak rapidly. To correct this and establish a desirable rate of speaking for all of us, we read slowly in unison. Short selections of poetry or prose are copied on a chalk board. As we read these we try to give each word its own beauty and meaning so as to break the habit of running them together into one unintelligible utterance. These same selections are used for individual practice in speaking loudly.

The member of the class who has most difficulty with breath control also has the most difficulty in speaking loudly. For him we emphasize deep breaths before starting each sentence. Sometimes we select a reading for words which require a coordinated use of all the speaking muscles for good enunciation. "Twinkle, twinkle, little star" is a favorite for this. Other expressive words are "squash," "squabble," "quack." Sometimes we substitute one of these for the words of a familiar song and sing them.

Our patients must learn to apply these techniques of speech improvement in their daily conversation, so we talk together. At the start of a class, members like to report what kind of a night they have had, comment on a TV program or a special meeting in the chapel, and tell of any special events in their lives, such as an outing with their families. Sometimes we use almost the entire class period for conversation, selecting one subject for our talk. These conversation days are morale-boosters when the class is weary and frustrated by exercises. As the classes continue, they will probably involve more conversation sessions, since the basic exercises and drills have been fairly well established.

Classes run from 20 to 30 minutes and are held three times a week. It is important to check a few details before starting. Has everyone had a drink of water before coming to class? (Some antiparkinson drugs dry the mouth.) Have dentures been secured with dental cream? Is there a supply of Kleenex readily available for those who drool?

The Home's administrator was the first person to comment about results: "What have you done with Joe? The other day he was in the office and I could understand him." Joe was the professor. Several weeks later one of Ray's visitors remarked, "Other times I couldn't understand him, but tonight I could understand everything he said." Ray was the junior high school teacher. Of Ruth, the governess, several nurses said that the classes were helping her.

Putting these statements together in this way gives the impression that the class has been a huge success, but it has taken many weeks to earn these few compliments. Improvement has been slow and inconsistent. Joe or Ray or Ruth speak well today, but articulate poorly tomorrow. Any number of factors affect their speech: a poor night's sleep, arthritic pain, an emotional upset before class.

Each member responds in his own way. Ruth practices the exercises in her room between classes. Attending classes is the event of the week for her. Joe seems to enjoy the attention of the classroom, more than the discipline of speaking slowly and clearly. Ray submits to exercises reluctantly, but becomes alive and cooperative in conversation. As we work with them, we try to give each one a sense of worth as a person and thus make their lives more enjoyable.

Section III Disorders Requiring Neurosurgery or Acute Care

Underlying conditions can alter the neurosurgical patient's postoperative course and require special attention. In this section, the complex care required for such patients is outlined. The acute care of patients with a variety of neuromuscular problems is also described. The principles of care identified in these articles can be applied to the nursing of patients with other, similar disorders.

A Delicate Balance: Managing Chronic Airway Obstruction in a Neurosurgical Patient

GWEN J. STEPHENS • MICKEY C. PARSONS

The patient had a high level of preoperative anxiety and so was tranquilized. But the tranquilized patient with CAO encounters serious breathing problems.

Ms. E., a 47-year-old woman, was admitted to the University of Colorado Medical Center for removal of a cerebellopontine angle (CPA) tumor.

For 10 years she had had tinnitus and a progressive hearing loss in her right ear. More recently, she had experienced ataxia and episodes of vertigo and had noted finger incoordination which interfered with her favorite pastime, sewing. On the basis of a number of procedures—tomography, skull films, cerebrospinal fluid analysis, audiometry, brain scan, and pneumoencephalogram—Ms. E. had been diagnosed as having a large (about 2 cm.) right acoustic nerve tumor.

Most acoustic nerve tumors arise from the vestibular branch of the eighth cranial nerve and are discrete and encapsulated. As they enlarge, they compress and distort cranial nerves V (trigeminal), VII (facial), and VIII (acoustic), as well as displace and indent the parts of the pons and cerebellum in their vicinity. The most common symptoms are deaf-

GWEN JONES STEPHENS, R.N., Ph.D., is an associate professor and chairman, Graduate Medical-Surgical Nursing, University of Colorado Medical Center School of Nursing, Denver. MICKEY C. PARSONS, R.N., M.S., is assistant director, nursing service, University of Colorado Medical Center Hospital, and assistant professor, University of Colorado Medical Center School of Nursing, Denver, Colorado.

ness, tinnitus, disturbed equilibrium, and later, as the tumor enlarges, headache from the increased intracranial pressure.

The decision concerning surgery for removal of this neurinoma was difficult because Ms. E. also had chronic airway obstruction (CAO). This was due to her alpha-l-antitrypsin deficiency emphysema with cor pulmonale. Pulmonary complications are a common cause of postoperative mortality in neurosurgical patients with chronic airway obstruction. The combination of diminished lung recoil with airway obstruction, caused by bronchial edema, inflammation, and copious secretions, leads to marked hypoxemia and hypercapnia.

Alpha-l-antitrypsin emphysema apparently stems from a genetically determined reduction of alpha-l-antitrypsin, an important plasma globulin. In an acute lung infection, certain leukocytes release proteolytic enzymes. The action of these leukoproteases is antagonized by plasma antitrypsins. However, in the antitrypsin-deficient patient, the enzymes cause hydrolysis and destruction of both lung capillaries and parenchyma. The long-term consequences are a decline in elastic recoil, alveolar overdistention and destruction, and the partial obliteration of pulmonary capillary circulation. The arterial blood gases are further compromised by the elevated O_2 consumption and CO_2 production that result from the increased work of breathing.

The mechanism of cor pulmonale in CAO is complicated, and not all of the causative factors are known. Pulmonary vasoconstriction probably occurs in response to both the chronic arterial hypoxia and the acidemia correlated with periods of increased CO_2 retention. This vasoconstriction leads to pulmonary hypertension. Destruction of the normal alveolar structure obliterates large portions of the pulmonary capillary bed, which worsens the pulmonary artery hypertension. The consequence is a chronically increased workload on the right ventricle, producing right ventricular hypertrophy. Thus, both structural change (pulmonary capillary destruction) and functional change (pulmonary capillary constriction) produce cor pulmonale and systemic venous congestion in the patient with emphysema and bronchitis.

BEGINNING DIFFICULTIES

Although Ms. E. had been following a pulmonary rehabilitation program at home, she still experienced episodes of orthopnea, dyspnea on exertion, and ankle edema. Her home program had included continuous nasal oxygen at 3 to 4 l./min. oxtriphylline (a xanthine bronchodilator), digoxin, furosemide (Lasix), potassium supplements, and chlordiazepoxide (Librium) for chronic anxiety.

On admission to the hospital, Ms. E. was extremely anxious over the projected operation, so the Librium dosage was increased.

Over the next few days she became increasingly dyspneic, cyanotic, and lethargic, with evidence of worsening pulmonary congestion. Her temperature rose to 38.8 C. with chills. Measurement of arterial blood gases (ABG) on 5 l./in. nasal oxygen revealed PaO_2 48, $PaCO_2$ 75, and pH 7.30. She was in acute respiratory distress and a chest x-ray showed a lower left lobe infiltrate. Her white count was elevated and sputum cultures grew *Pseudomonas*.

The medical and nursing staff speculated that her worsening pulmonary status resulted from oversedation with Librium. The increase in this tranquilizer had decreased her efforts to maintain adequate pulmonary hygiene through productive coughing, deep breathing, and general physical activity. Respiratory depression with decreased secretion clearance led to acute bronchitis and pneumonia.

Ms. E.'s nursing care at this time included intense bronchial hygiene. This consisted of intermittent positive pressure breathing (IPPB) treatments with a bronchial dilator followed by warm nebulized water through a face tent for 15 minues, and postural drainage with percussion and vigorous coughing every two hours to clear pulmonary secretions. Her physical activity included frequent position changes in bed and sitting in a chair at least four times a day. The physicians ordered chloramphenicol (Chloromycetin) 4 Gm./day, although this is not often the drug of choice for *Pseudomonas*.

With this management, her respiratory status gradually improved, although she complained of frequent severe headaches. The staff speculated that while part of this discomfort could be caused by pressure from the tumor, it was probably also induced by high levels of CO_2 retention, which leads to dilation of cerebral vessels and cerebrovascular congestion.

We noted that when Ms. E. was sufficiently active the headache seemed to abate, suggesting that increased activity improved alveolar ventilation. Then, with relief of pain, she was more willing to cough productively and this, in turn, further improved her alveolar ventilation by clearing secretions from the airways.

After two weeks, the neurosurgeons and pulmonary medicine physicians thought that Ms. E.'s respiratory status had cleared enough for surgery to be reasonably safe. A right suboccipital craniectomy was performed and a large acoustic neurinoma was removed, with unavoidable sacrifice of the right cranial nerves VII and VIII.

The surgeons placed an intraventricular catheter through a burr hole for monitoring her intracranial pressure (ICP) postoperatively and removing cerebrospinal fluid in the event that acute hydrocephalus developed from cerebral edema. This monitor remained in place 24 hours. The difficulties during surgery, in addition to cranial nerve sacrifice, were a hypotensive episode in which her systolic blood pressure dropped to 70 mm. Hg early in the operation, bleeding from a cerebellar artery, and the extremely delicate maneuvers necessary to dislodge the large tumor from its intimate relation to the right pontine area.

Postoperatively, Ms. E. was returned to the surgical intensive therapy unit. She had an endotracheal tube in place and was on a volume ventilator. Her vital sgns, ABGs, and mental status were satisfactory. Her posterior cranial nerves—IX (glossopharyngeal), X (vagus), XI (spinal accessory), and XII (hypoglossal)—were functioning satisfactorily. Their functions are checked by testing the patient's gag reflex and having her swallow, shrug her shoulders, and extend her tongue. Her ICP was a normal 4 mm. Hg. That evening and the following day her ECG showed some premature ventricular contractions. These were controlled with lidocaine, but their cause was not determined.

During Ms. E.'s second postoperative day, she was taken off the ventilator and placed on a T-piece for 20-minute periods with frequent assessment of her pulse, blood pressure, respiratory rate, tidal volumes, and ABGs. A T-piece is a plastic tube in the shape of a T. The perpendicular portion fits over the endotracheal tube; oxygen tubing is attached to one portion of the cross piece and the expired air can exit from the other openings.

She was able to communicate with the staff by writing. Because her condition remained satisfactory, her endotracheal tube was removed 48 hours after surgery. She received O_2 continuously at 6 l./min. through nasal prongs and 40 percent O_2 through a nebulizer face tent intermittently.

At 3:30 A.M. of her third postoperative day, Ms. E. became markedly agitated. As we approached her bedside, we saw that her left arm and leg were tonically flexed and that subsequently she exhibited bilateral clonic movements. This seizure was accompanied by cyanosis and respiratory arrest. The physician inserted an endotracheal tube promptly and she then began breathing spontaneously. Within 10 minutes of the seizure, she was awake and able to respond to verbal commands. We assumed that she had suffered no brain damage affecting higher mental functions.

To rule out acute hydrocephalus as a cause of the seizure, the physician attempted to insert a cannula into the lateral ventricle through the posterior burr hole. Failure to locate the ventricle indicated that the ventricles were not dilated and, therefore, that elevated ICP probably was not the cause of her seizure. We speculated that gradually decreasing tidal volumes with increasing cerebral hypoxia had induced the convulsion. Consequently, we planned to ventilate her mechanically for the rest of the night.

Ms. E. became markedly agitated, however, and if she had remained on the ventilator, she would have required sedation. Therefore we left her on the T-piece and determined her vital signs, respiratory rate, tidal volume, and ABGs frequently throughout the night. We gave diphenylhydantoin (Dilantin) to suppress further seizure discharge.

It is a well-established fact that generalized cerebral hypoxia may lead to periodic seizures. Extreme alveolar hypoventilation causes arterial hypoxemia. This decreases cerebral oxygen supply to levels that may cause spontaneous neural firing. The symptoms of cerebral hypoxia may range from confusion and agitation to loss of consciousness, myoclonic convulsions, focal motor seizures, or generalized grand mal tonic-clonic seizures.

A focal epileptogenic lesion may be produced originally by hypoxic neuron damage from a seizure occurring during cardiopulmonary arrest. Then, once such a group of abnormally excitable neurons has developed, additional periods of hypoxia during acute alveolar hypoventilation may trigger repeated convulsive episodes. The result is an extension of pathological neuron excitability and increased seizure susceptibility as a response to further arterial hypoxemia.

It is not unusual for such hypoxic seizures to occur more frequently at night. A patient tends to maintain better arterial oxygen tensions during the day. During sleep, the $PaCO_2$ level rises and O_2 tension falls because there is a decrease in general sensory input and nonspecific neural drive to the respiratory centers and a fall in muscular activity with a resulting decline in catecholamines. These physiological changes lead to nocturnal hypercapnia, which causes a compensatory renal-bicarbonate retention (metabolic alkalosis) that acts as a further respiratory depressant. Eventually, hypoxemia reaches a level that triggers neuron discharge in the epileptogenic focus.

Treatment is mainly symptomatic. The patient is given anticonvulsants to suppress the excessive neuronal firing. Those medications known to be respiratory depressants must be avoided. All measures possible to improve alveolar ventilation must be taken.

During the following afternoon, it became evident from her anxiety and discomfort that Ms. E. was not tolerating the endotracheal tube well. Since her respiratory status was now adequate, the endotracheal tube was removed and she was given O_2 through nasal prongs at 3 l./min., and 70 percent O_2 by face tent. An hour later her ABG analysis showed pH 7.42, pO_2 75, and pCO_2 53, which we considered satisfactory.

Two days later, which was her fifth postoperative day, Ms. E. began having generalized seizures. The first was accompanied by extreme cyanosis and respiratory arrest. The second episode occurred while we were bag-breathing her. She was again intubated, but this time with great difficulty. Her blood gases after the intubation and while being ventilated with a self-inflating bag were pH 7.22, pO_2 50, and CO_2 75. She was placed on a volume ventilator which was set for an FIO_2 (fraction of inspired oxygen) of 0.6, tidal volume of 700, and respiratory rate of 15.

Ms. E. had two more grand mal seizures, which were treated with I.V. diazepam (Valium). The physician increased her dosage of Dilantin and added phenobarbital to her anticonvulsant regimen. Four hours later she persisted in status epilepticus although now the seizures were confined to her left side.

At this time, the neurosurgeons were concerned that these seizures might be caused by posterior fossa bleeding or some other mass lesion. They ordered an immediate angiogram which appeared to be within normal limits. The neuroradiologist thought that her hypoventilation was associated with a bradycardia which in turn was leading to impaired cerebral arterial filling and thus, again, to cerebral ischemia and hypoxia. The poor cerebral oxygenation could be initiating the generalized seizures. The doctors concluded that cerebral hypoxia, rather than a mass lesion or elevated intracranial pressure, was causing the seizures.

Ms. E. had generalized seizures most of that fifth day which culminated in muscle flaccidity on her left side. Toward evening, her convulsions became less frequent. She was more alert and could move her left hand very slightly.

PHYSIOLOGICAL ALTERATIONS

In a patient like Ms. E. who is having repeated acute respiratory failure superimposed on severe CAO, there are various abnormalities in blood gases, acid-base balance, and electrolytes. These patients generally have problems with chronic electrolyte and acid-base abnormalities, chronic alterations of the respiratory center and associated reflexes, and acute acid-base shifts in systemic and central nervous system fluid spaces.

CHRONIC ELECTROLYTE AND ACID-BASE ABNORMALITIES A patient with chronically elevated $PaCO_2$ from CAO may have a normal plasma pH because of the renal compensatory mechanism in respiratory acidosis. In this situation, the kidneys eliminate hydrogen ions and reabsorb corresponding amounts of bicarbonate. A chronic metabolic alkalosis can result which can worsen the patient's respiratory status by causing depression of the respiratory centers and the reflex respiratory response to CO_2 mediated by the chemoreceptors.

Patients with this type of renal metabolic alkalosis are sometimes given acetazolamide (Diamox) to facilitate kidney elimination of bicarbonate. Acetazolamide suppresses the enzyme carbonic anhydrase. This enzyme makes hydrogen ions available for excretion at the renal tubular cells by catalyzing the reaction: $H_2O + CO_2 \rightleftarrows H_2CO_3 \rightleftarrows H^+ + HCO_3^-$. By inhibiting this enzyme, H^+ excretion and HCO_3^- resorption by the kidney are decreased. A slight metabolic acidosis results and plasma pH returns to a more normal level.

In a patient like Ms. E., this would have two favorable consequences: less respiratory depression and hence an improved alveolar ventilation and a decreased neural susceptibility to seizure discharge. A mild acidosis tends to inhibit spontaneous depolarization of neural epileptogenic foci.

Electrolyte and acid-base abnormalities are often made worse in CAO patients when diuretics are used to treat coexising cor pulmonale. Diuretics tend to promote chloride loss and therefore add to the renal compensatory alkalosis. Diuretics produce this effect by stimulating the renal distal tubule cation-exchange site, where sodium ion (Na^+) resorption takes place in exchange for H^+ and potassium ion (K^+) elimination.

The H^+ and K^+ loss leads to increased bicarbonate regeneration, worsening the alkalemia and hypokalemia. A low blood potassium enhances digitalis toxicity, impairs respiratory muscle function, and depresses myocardial contractility. Therefore, most diuretics must be used cautiously in these patients and plasma electrolyte and pH values must be monitored carefully.

Conversely, the CAO patient with cor pulmonale often responds favorably to diuretics: the ABG status improves because the diuretic has helped decrease the excess fluid congestion in the lungs. Lung compliance increases, the work of breathing decreases, and alveolar ventilation improves.

CHRONIC ALTERATIONS OF THE RESPIRATORY CENTERS AND ASSOCIATED REFLEXES In normal individuals, low plasma-oxygen tension stimulates the peripheral chemoreceptors to increase ventilation. In chronic hypoxemia, however, ventilatory response to lowered PaO_2 is depressed. There also is evidence that chronic hypoxemia depresses the sensitivity of the repiratory centers to all physiological mechanisms that normally stimulate it.

In addition, prolonged hypercapnia blunts ventilatory response to increased CO_2 levels, both directly at the respiratory centers and reflexly through the chemoreceptors. For these reasons, the CAO patient with chronic severely abnormal blood gases (hypoxia and hypercapnia) relies heavily on hypoxic drive to maintain ventilation, although this response is often attenuated. It is this hypoxic drive which makes it hazardous to give these patients uncontrolled O_2 therapy; the elevated PaO_2 may remove hypoxic ventilatory stimulation and result in cardiopulmonary arrest.

ACUTE ACID-BASE SHIFTS RESULTING FROM ACUTE RESPIRATORY FAILURE
Acute respiratory failure readily occurs with acute bronchitis or pneumonia or pharmacological respiratory depression with sedatives or tranquilizers. The patient's pulmonary status deteriorates; there is acute carbon dioxide retention and a marked fall in PaO_2. Cerebral hypoxia may impair the patient's brain function.

In addition, the rapid rise in $PaCO_2$ will cause an acute respiratory acidemia. Carbon dioxide crosses brain capillary membranes with ease. Thus a marked increase in $PaCO_2$ will cause a corresponding rapid fall in pH of cerebrospinal fluid (CSF) and brain extracellular fluid (ECF). This CSF acidosis may be associated with marked impairment of brain function.

When plasma pH falls below 7.20, systemic hypotension, myocardial irritability, and cardiac arrest may occur. These are complicated by the simultaneous hypoxia and hypercapnia, which themselves induce cardiac arrhythmias. The myocardium, especially in the cor pulmonate patient receiving digitalis, is more prone to develop toxic arrhythmias during severe hypoxemia. The arrhythmias may result in a decreased cerebral perfusion and brain ischemia. The result may be a triggering of hypoxic seizures.

Bicarbonate crosses the blood-brain barrier more slowly than CO_2. Shortly after the brain pH is sharply lowered in respiratory failure, bicarbonate equilibrates between brain ECF and systemic ECF, and the pH of the brain returns to more normal levels. If the patient in respiratory failure is then placed on mechanical ventilation and his $PaCO_2$ declines too rapidly, CO_2 leaves brain ECF and CSF along the now reversed gradient. Brain alkalemia may occur, resulting in further impairment in neurological function.

CONTEMPORARY NURSING SERIES

ESTABLISHING ADEQUATE VENTILATION

Ten days postoperatively, Ms. E. showed marked improvement; she responded readily to verbal stimuli and mouthed words understandably. Her left hand was becoming stronger and she could sit up on the edge of the bed. She tolerated tube feedings well. We began weaning her from the ventilator.

Weaning was a difficult process. We started by placing her on 40 percent O_2 through a T-piece attached to her tracheostomy tube. We established baseline ABGs while she was on the ventilator and then assessed her ABGs, vital signs, tidal volume, skin color, and anxiety at frequent intervals while she was off the ventilator. She could tolerate being off only 15 minutes initially, but the free periods lengthened gradually. She required constant observation because there was no consistency in lengths of time she could breathe on her own. Suddenly her tidal volume would decline to about 100, her respiratory rate would rise to 40, and mechanical ventilation would become necessary.

Throughout this period, she required vigorous respiratory nursing care —suctioning at least hourly and postural drainage with chest percussion every two to four hours. She received IPPB treatments with a bronchodilator every four hours for 15 minutes. Eventually she could breathe on her own for up to 16 hours. Despite her gradual physical improvement, Ms. E. periodically became extremely anxious and frustrated, at times belligerent. She wanted to be better "right now"; she wanted all the tubes out immediately. She pulled out her Foley catheter and nasogastric tube. Occasionally we had to restrain her arms. We tried to help her cope with her emotional problems by letting her make decisions about her care when possible.

Finally she was able to sit in a chair 30 minutes twice a day and could take oral fluids. She began walking while we ventilated her with a self-inflating bag. She was beginning to have a sense of hope for survival and started to talk about her fears concerning chronic invalidism, the completeness of her recovery, and whether she would be a burden to her husband and teen-aged children.

Within a week her tracheostomy tube was replaced with a Kistner button. This button makes it possible to keep the opening in the tissue from closing over. Then, if a tracheostomy tube must be replaced, it can be done quickly and easily. The staff can keep this button at an open position or begin to close it off to help the patient reestablish her own breathing pattern.

Ms. E. continued on oxygen by nasal prongs at 5 l./min. with a 40 percent oxygen face tent. When she could tolerate having the Kistner button closed for two days, we transferred her to the ward.

The next day, the ward staff noted that Ms. E. had a great deal of sputum, shortness of breath, and perioral and nailbed cyanosis. And, again, at 3:30 A.M., she became very dyspneic and had an irregular heart beat that culminated in cardiopulmonary arrest. Whether this was preceded by a seizure is not known.

Ms. E. received two I.V. boluses of sodium bicarbonate, was intubated, ventilated with 40 percent oxygen with a self-inflating bag, and suctioned. This brought forth copious bloody secretions. Her pupils were fully dilated. As these emergency measures were in progress, ABGs were drawn and showed her pH to be 7.11, PaO_2 40, and $PaCO_2$ 64. She was transferred to the ICU, where she stabilized and did not require mechanical ventilation.

The following day her mental status appeared satisfactory, but at 1:30 the next morning, she had convulsive activity which began with left focal twitching of her eye, mouth, face, and hand. This progressed to complete rigidity and a grand mal seizure, followed by respiratory arrest.

The immediate cause of this recurrence of seizure activity was discussed at length by the medical and nursing staff. Possible causes included pulmonary obstruction from a buildup of secretions with resulting hypoxia (her oxygen was off at the time of the seizure), an IPPB treatment with Bronkosol just before her seizure, and a run of ventricular tachycardia during this treatment.

A possible sequence of events might have been hypoxia leading to an arrhythmia that was triggered or made worse by the bronchodilator; then decreased cardiac output that caused a decline in cerebral perfusion; and, finally, cerebral hypoxia which triggered susceptible epileptogenic foci. These foci could have been a residual from her neurosurgery or from the previous hypoxic brain damage during earlier seizures.

Following this arrest, Ms. E. could be aroused only slowly and her level of consciousness was impaired. She had mental confusion intermittently.

CONTROLLING SEIZURES UPSET VENTILATION

The medical and nursing staffs found themselves in a perplexing double bind; controlling her seizures with anticonvulsants made her lethargic to somnolent. This depressed her rate and depth of respirations, which produced a fall in alveolar ventilation and then cerebral hypoxia and seizures. But decreasing the neural depressants resulted in a marked increase in excitability and spontaneous neural discharge, probably with generalization throughout the brain. This would promote further hypoxic brain damage.

The decision was to decrease her Bronkosol dosage for future IPPB treatments and to increase her Dilantin. To help clear her pulmonary secretions and ameliorate arterial hypoxemia, we encouraged fluids to 3,000 cc. By keeping her well hydrated, her secretions were thinned and therefore easier to remove.

About 40 days after her operation, Ms. E.'s condition had stabilized enough that the Kistner button could be removed. The physicians commented that apparently, as long as Ms. E. continued to ventilate reasonably well, the irritable brain foci responsible for the convulsions would not be triggered.

Unfortunately, the following day after a 10-minute IPPB treatment, Ms. E. had three generalized seizures, accompanied by cyanois and respiratory arrest. Her pH was 7.02 and her PCO_2 94. She was profoundly somnolent and confused following this episode and had frequent PVCs. Her electroenchephalogram was grossly abnormal: diffuse persistent slowly over the right hemisphere with slow and disorganized activity from the left.

From the EEG and other neurological findings, it appeared that hypoxia from inadequate alveolar ventilation was responsible for the seizures, abnormal EEG, somnolence, and mental confusion. She had a true metabolic encephalopathy or organic brain syndrome on an hypoxic basis.

THE FINAL PRIORITY

In the next several months, Ms. E.'s mental, respiratory, and cardiac condition followed a downhill course. She was in and out of the ICU for acute respiratory failure and was frequently hospitalized at the university psychiatric facility for suicidal depression, agitation, and profound confusion. Her anxiety worsened her respiratory status because she abandoned all attempts to carry out pulmonary hygiene. Seizures continued frequently, many leaving a postictal left-sided paresis.

With the help of her pulmonary medicine physician, Ms. E. and her family finally decided that the most sensible and kind course was to not resuscitate her when the next inevitable respiratory arrest occurred. All of them saw further heroic measures as ill advised and in fact cruel.

Ms. E. died of respiratory failure in a nursing home six months after her surgery. The major autopsy findings were severe bilateral emphysema with focal fibrosis and chronic bronchitis, right ventricular hypertrophy, and pulmonary artery atherosclerosis. There was focal necrosis of the pons and some necrosis of the right temporal lobe tip. The pathologist thought that these changes resembled hypoxic ischemic ones rather than aftereffects of the tumor surgery. He found no evidence of tumor recurrence and, with respect to her seizures, he was unable to locate a distinct focus. However, neural membrane physiological alterations in excitability threshold adequate to produce even severe and recurrent seizures are not generally distinguishable by methods presently available.

Our struggle in Ms. E.'s behalf was a long and perplexing effort to maneuver her safely though the delicate balance between maintaining adequate ventilation and controlling her seizures. Despite the accumulated knowledge about care, there is a point when we all must recognize the time to give up the heroics out of respect for the person. That, too, is good care.

BIBLIOGRAPHY

FILLEY, G. F. *Acid-Base and Blood Gas Regulation.* Philadelphia, Lea and Febiger, 1971.

GASTAUT, HENRI, AND BROUGHTON, R. J. *Epeliptic Seizures: Clinical and Electrographic Features, Diagnosis and Treatment.* Springfield, Ill., Charles C Thomas, Publisher, 1972.

GASTAUT, HENRI, AND OTHERS. *The Physiopathogenesis of the Epilepsies.* Springfield, Ill., Charles C Thomas, Publisher, 1969.

HUDAK, C. M., AND OTHERS. *Critical Care Nursing.* Philadelphia, J. B. Lippincott Co., 1973.

JOHNSTON, R. F., ED. *Pulmonary Care.* New York, Grune and Stratton, 1973.

MITTMAN, CHARLES, ED. *Pulmonary Emphysema and Proteolysis.* Symposium held at the City of Hope Medical Center, Duarte, Calif., Jan. 1971 (City of Hope Symposium Series) New York, Academic Press, 1972.

NIEDERMEYER, ERNST, *Compendium of the Epilepsies,* Springfield, Ill., Charles C Thomas, Publisher, 1973.

PETTY, T. L. *Intensive and Rehabilitative Respiratory Care.* 2d ed. Philadelphia, Lea and Febiger, 1974.

PLUM, FRED, AND POSNER, J. B. EDS. *The Diagnosis of Stupor and Coma.* 2d ed. (Contemporary Neurology Series No. 6) Philadelphia, F. A. Davis Co., 1972.

POOL, J. L., AND OTHERS. *Acoustic Nerve Tumors: Early Diagnosis and Treatment.* 2d ed. Springfield, Ill., Charles C Thomas, Publisher, 1970.

SCHMIDT, R. P., AND WILDER, B. J. *Epilepsy: A Clinical Textbook.* (Contemporary Neurology Series No. 2) Phila., F. A. Davis Co., 1968.

Hypophysectomy for Diabetic Retinopathy

SHARON M. STOWE

Diabetes which is resistant to diet and insulin therapy is often easier to control—and retinal deterioration slowed— if certain pituitary hormones are prevented from being excreted by destruction of the pituitary gland.

For a few patients with diabetic retinopathy, hypophysectomy, or removal of the pituitary gland, is the palliative procedure of choice to slow or halt their progressive blindness(1).

Four of the anterior pituitary hormones—corticotropin, thyrotropin, luteotropin, and growth—have, in susceptible patients, a diabetogenic effect. Interrupting the production and dissemination of these hormones, by hypophysectomy, and replacing them with chemical substitutes in controlled amounts have arrested some patients' retinal damage and made their diabetes easier to control(2).

Ms. R., a 19-year-old, single, Puerto Rican girl, was one of my patients who had an hypophysectomy. She had a history of repeated retinal hemorrhages, progressive loss of vision for two years prior to admission, and diabetes which was refractory to a well-supervised and frequently adjusted regimen of diet and insulin. She was a good candidate for hypophysectomy because her renal and cardiac functions were within normal limits and because she wanted very much to live a more normal life and preserve her remaining vision.

To plan and carry out the best possible care for Ms. R., I needed to

---

MS. STOWE, *who is a clinical nurse specialist in Neurology and Neurosurgery at the Veterans Administration Hospital, Bronx, N.Y., is a graduate of the Kaiser Foundation School of Nursing, Oakland, Calif. She earned a B.S. degree at the University of Washington, Seattle, and an M.A. degree in nursing education at New York University, N.Y.*

know the cause of diabetic retinopathy, the relationship of the pituitary gland to the diabetic process, methods commonly used to ablate the pituitary gland, and the signs and symptoms of hypopituitarism and how these can be relieved or prevented. I also needed to be able to prepare this patient for permanent changes in her lifestyle which would occur as a result of hypophysectomy. In addition, I needed to learn from the patient herself how she practiced her diabetic therapy, what she knew about diabetes and about her reduced vision, and what she understood about an hypophysectomy.

Davis and others believe that diabetic retinopathy begins with capillary changes in the retina, which are related to the faulty carbohydrate metabolism and oxidation which are part of the diabetic syndrome. The retinal capillaries and terminal arterioles become narrowed and/or obliterated with gradually increasing ischemia, hemorrhage, exudation, and edema which causes necrosis of retinal tissue. Such unchecked pathology gradually results in irreversible blindness(3).

RELATIONSHIP OF THE PITUITARY (HYPOPHYSEAL) GLAND TO THE DIABETIC PROCESS The pituitary gland is considered the master gland of the endocrine system. Through a negative feedback mechanism, it regulates hormone production of the thyroid, testes, and ovaries. The hormones of the pituitary are believed to have an effect also on the thymus, parathyroid, and pancreatic glands. Whether the effect is direct or indirect is unknown at present. The pituitary is centrally located under the frontal lobe of the brain, within the sella turcica under the branches of the optic chiasm. The hypophyseal stalk connects the pituitary to the hypothalamus.

The pars intermedia divides the gland into two sections: the adenohypophysis, or anterior pituitary, and the neurohypophysis, or posterior pituitary. Six hormones are secreted by the adenohypophysis: luteotropic hormone (LH), luteinizing hormone (LTH), follicle stimulating hormone (FSH), thyrotropin, growth hormone, and corticotropin (ACTH). The neurohypophysis secretes antidiuretic hormone (ADH or vasopressin) and oxytocin.

Of the six hormones secreted by the adenohypophysis, only one, growth hormone, acts directly on almost all tissues. The other five have specific target glands: the adrenal cortex, the thymus, the thyroid gland, pancreatic glands, and the gonads. The two hormones secreted by the neurohypophysis, oxytocin and ADH, are manufactured by specialized nerve cells in the hypothalamus. The posterior pituitary is thus regarded as a "storage organ" for oxytocin and ADH(4).

Oxytocin promotes contraction of the pregnant uterus and is responsible for milk let-down during lactation; antidiuretic hormone affects the collecting tubules of the kidney.

Antidiuretic hormone plays an important part in normal fluid and electrolyte balance and, therefore, its loss is a grave consideration in surgery of the pituitary. This hormone increases the water permeability of the collecting tubules of the kidney. It is secreted when body fluids become highly concentrated. Without ADH a person can lose large amounts of water while initially retaining electrolytes.

In diabetes insipidus, a condition in which ADH is either absent or lacking, a person drinks large amounts of water to replace the fluid lost, and thus "washes out" the electrolytes. In conditions of stress, or when fluid and salt are not readily available, a person may experience electrolyte imbalance, dehydration, and death.

Four anterior pituitary hormones have a diabetogenic effect. Growth hormone reduces carbohydrate metabolism within all body cells, increases the amount of glycogen in the cells, and reduces the amount of glucose normally taken up by the cells. Growth hormone, therefore, raises the blood glucose concentration above normal. Corticotropin, thyrotropin, and luteotropin act on the adrenal cortex and thyroid and mammary glands, to indirectly increase the rate of gluconeogenesis. Elimination of these effects is part of the rationale for doing hypophysectomies on patients with diabetes that is resistant to diet and insulin therapy(5).

SIGNS AND SYMPTOMS OF HYPOPITUITARISM The physiologic effects of hypophysectomy are those of induced hypopituitarism. The most dramatic and rapidly occurring effect is diabetes insipidus due to loss of ADH. In addition to excessive fluid loss through the kidneys and a corresponding excessive thirst, the urine is noticeable pale and waterlike and has a low specific gravity. If diabetes insipidus is unchecked, the patient soon shows mental and physical signs of electrolyte imbalance.

Another result of induced hypopituitarism is adrenocortical insufficiency due to loss of ACTH. This effect is demonstrated by hypoglycemia (which is especially apt to occur in a person with diabetes if insulin dosage is not carefully adjusted following hypophysectomy), low serum sodium, and elevated potassium and blood urea nitrogen levels. Patients with secondary adrenocortical insufficiency have a low physiological stress tolerance(6).

Other effects, which are slower to occur and may be more insidious, are hypothyroidism and hypogonadism. Hypothyroidism is seen in adults as myxedema. Hypogonadism in the adult is demonstrated by loss of libido and potency; in adult females, by a gradual loss of menses and resulting sterility. Both males and females may lose secondary sex characteristics.

METHODS TO ABLATE THE PITUITARY GLAND Removal or destruction of the pituitary gland can be done in various ways: heavy particle pituitary suppression; implantation of Yttrium 90; coagulation of the pituitary gland with radiofrequency; cryohypophysectomy; and total or partial removal using a cranial frontal lobe approach(7).

In the transphenoidal microsurgical procedure, the patient is given endotracheal induction anesthesia. Under the upper lip a midline incision is made to start the rhinoseptal approach into the sella turcica. When the pituitary gland is adequately seen, it is dissected from its stalk until it is entirely removed. The sella turcica is packed with muscle or fat from the thigh, the sphenoid sinus is packed with silastic medical adhesive, and the sella window is closed with a cartilaginous graft, usually from the nasal septum. All of this packing and grafting is necessary to prevent leakage of cerebral spinal fluid. A large external incision is not necessary because visualization is accomplished with a surgical microscope, an image amplifier, and a television screen(8).

The primary advantages of this technique are that a large external incision is unnecessary, there is no need to shave the patient's head. and trauma to surrounding brain structure is minimal. However, it is difficult to seal the sella turcica tightly enough to prevent leakage of cerebral spinal fluid and it is difficult to see, even with a microscope and amplifier, whether the stalk is being sectioned high enough so that no portion of the gland is left in the sella turcica. (If even a few cells are left behind, the gland may continue to function.)

The surgeons planned to totally remove Ms. R's pituitary with a cranial frontal lobe approach. In this procedure, a scalp incision is made approximately 1 inch behind the hairline. Then, an opening is made into the right frontal bone and the cerebral spinal fluid drained. After this, a dehydrating agent (hypertonic saline) may be given to reduce the size of the brain, the right frontal lobe is elevated and the pituitary divided at the diaphragma sellae. The pituitary gland is then removed by successive use of curettement, suction, and abrasive swabbing, followed by electrocoagulation or the application of Zenker's Solution to the cavity of the sella(9).

This technique assures total removal of the gland, thereby preventing its regrowth with remanufacture of hypophyseal hormones. Further, there is visual assurance that the sella turcica is intact and not likely to leak cerebrospinal fluid. The chief disadvantage of this technique is that the patient must undergo the physical and emotional stress of a craniotomy.

MEDICAL MANAGEMENT OF HYPOPITUITARISM Following hypophysectomy there must be careful evaluation of the patient's hormonal levels with replacement of hormones as necessary. Ms. R. needed to realize that she would need lifelong medical management. It was my responsibility to make sure she understood the benefits and consequences of this surgery, and that she would be a willing and active participant in her therapy.

PREOPERATIVE PREPARATION

During my initial contact with Ms. R., I found she was very willing to talk not only about her past, but also about her present physical problems and the impending surgery. Although she required assistance with reading assignments, she was doing quite well as a college freshman. She also had acquired a good knowledge of diabetes through frequent visits to various endocrine and metabolism clinics. She told me what she had been told about the expected effects of the surgery. She knew a hypophysectomy would not "cure" diabetes but would help her to control it, and, hopefully, arrest the retinopathy. We then discussed the what, when, why, and how of hormone replacement therapy. She believed all the effects of surgery would be worth the trouble if it preserved her remaining sight.

I began the next day by explaining the purpose and procedures for some of the necessary laboratory tests and explained that I would be with her to guide her through each step of preparation. First of all, several 24-hour urine tests were required to ascertain normal follicle stimulating hormone and lutenizing hormone levels excreted in the urine. Ms. R. readily accepted responsibility for carrying out these tests, which she had done several times before at home.

During this assessment period, Ms. R. was encouraged to talk to other patients on the unit who had had hypophysectomies. Members of the nursing and medical staffs encouraged her questions. I explained in detail what would happen to her and what would be expected of her in the weeks following surgery, and she frequently practiced coughing and deep breathing.

Because Ms. R. had difficulty in seeing the levels on the collecting pitcher, I placed small pieces of adhesive tape at each 50 cc. level so that by counting down the tapes to the point where her finger became wet she could estimate fairly accurately the amount of urine she had voided.

Post-hypophysectomy patients frequently receive antidiuretic hormone, when they need it, by inhalation. They use a "snuffer," a small atomizer containing a capsule with 1 mgm. of dissicated ADH, which is very rapidly absorbed through the nasal mucosa. After Ms. R. had been shown how to use the snuffer, she repeated the demonstration, using a blank capsule, sniffing first through one nostril and then through the other. She learned that to benefit from the medication she must avoid blowing her nose or sneezing for several minutes after using the snuffer.

Two days before surgery, I reviewed again with Ms. R. just what she had been taught. She had become anxious about the surgery and I thought her anxiety could be reduced if she could ask questions about specific events. For example, when I reminded her that she would get a preanesthetic medication by an intravenous injection, and would soon be off in a deep sleep, she said, "Then I won't be awake during my operation, and I won't see the O.R.?"

"That's right," I said. "You'll be asleep throughout the whole procedure, and you'll wake up in the recovery room when it is all over."

"Oh, I'm so glad to know that! I was afraid I might wake up while they were still working on me."

She wanted to know when her head would be shaved. I explained this would be done after she was asleep, in the preanesthesia room, and that probably only a small area would be shaved. She seemed anxious about being seen this way so I told her, "No one except the doctor will see your head because, before you leave the operating room, you will have a hat on. I then showed her a Cushing helmet, and told her that it is applied like a cast and dried with a hair dryer. I explained that the hat is light when it is dry, that if it began to feel too tight it could be cut, and that the original hat would probably be changed in three or four days, and a second hat worn for about a week.

We discussed events that would occur in the recovery room and what would happen when she was brought back to her room—she might have a headache but could have medication to ease the pain when she asked for it, she would be rather drowsy for the rest of the day, and she might be disoriented to time. I reminded her that her parents and I would be with her throughout the day and evening to help her, that the day after the operation she would feel more awake and alert, and she would be helped to get out of bed, and would then begin to take care of herself, as she is used to doing, with the amount of assistance gradually decreasing as she got better.

Preoperative events went exactly as I had told Ms. R. She had had no food or fluids from midnight on, had slept fitfully, showered early, seen her parents at 7:00 A.M., and, at 7:30 A.M., the night nurse had given the preoperative medications. Around 8:00 A.M., while her parents remained in her room, I escorted her to the preanesthesia room, where the anesthesiologist was waiting for her.

Mr. and Mrs. R. had done their best to hide their apprehension and anxiety from their daughter, but they were frightened. When I returned from the operating room floor, I took them to the cafeteria for "coffee and comforting." I tried to tell them a little of what was happening to their daughter, but I'm sure they comprehended little. After a while they went back to their daughter's room to wait. The strange looking equipment which had been set up for postoperative care added to their anxiety. I explained the purpose of the wall suction, oxygen supply, the blood pressure machine, and the intermittent positive pressure machine. They appeared fearful when I mentioned the tracheostomy tray, but seemed relieved when I told them a tracheostomy would be done only if it was absolutely necessary to help their daughter breathe, and that it was rarely needed for patients with this type of surgery.

Because they would be very significant persons in their daughter's postoperative care, I felt it was important to prepare them for their role during this stressful period. "Be yourselves," I emphasized.

IMMEDIATE POSTOPERATIVE CARE Early in the afternoon, Ms. R. returned from the recovery room. She had been transferred from the operating table directly to her own bed to preclude the hazards of transfer from stretcher to bed. She had been placed with her head at the foot of the bed to prevent any accidental changing of the 30-degree elevation of her head. This elevation facilitates venous return, thereby helping to ease intracranial pressure and headache. She was drowsy, but arousable, and fully reacted. To her parents she looked dreadful, of course. Her head was covered by the white Cushing helmet with a silver-dollar-sized, bright-red blood spot slightly above the center of her forehead. The hair dryer bonnet, which only partially covered the helmet, did not help her appearance. Her eyelids, though not yet black and blue, were puffy and swollen, and she could open them only a fraction. A nurse had placed iced compresses over her eyelids to help reduce the swelling and discomfort. I encouraged Ms. R.'s parents to replace the compresses with others from a nearby bowl as often as they seemed to need changing.

Although any patient who has undergone general anesthesia needs close nursing observations, a patient who has had a craniotomy must be watched for specific neurological complications. Ms. R. was pale, restless, and irritable, but no more so than someone with a severe headache. Although she complained of headache, she slept lightly at intervals. Her blood pressure and pulse were within the preoperative range. Her shallow respirations were slightly more rapid than they had been preoperatively, but were regular. Her pupils were equal in size and both reacted well to light, indicating no increased intracranial pressure.

Ms. R.'s handgrips were equal and strong. Her ability to move both feet against resistance was the same as preoperatively. Both of these normal signs meant that she had no damage to the motor cortex. Although irritable, she understood and responded appropriately to all verbal directions. She was checked every 15 minutes for the first four hours, then every hour until, in the judgment of nurses and doctors, this was no longer necessary. The primary purpose of these observations was to detect intracranial bleeding, which increases intracranial pressure which, in turn, produces headache, increased blood pressure and decreased pulse rate, respiratory arrhythmia and change in the level of consciousness—lethargy, slow verbal responses, coma.

Although Ms. R. complained of headache, she was given aspirin only after her temperature had been checked rectally to determine if she had fever. Headache accompanied by fever could be indicative of meningitis; therefore, aspirin given indiscriminately might mask the signs of meningeal infection.

Ms. R. complained often about her head dressing: it felt too tight, and her skin itched where the dressing touched it. Also, she didn't like the hair dryer. The noise made it difficult for her to sleep comfortably.

After checking the Cushing helmet to make sure it was not constricting, I adjusted the chin strap to make it easier for her to swallow and to talk, and I tried cushioning the hair dryer to reduce the noise.

Ms. R. was worried about the intravenous needle in her hand; it hurt and she was afraid she might pull it out or disconnect it. I tried repositioning her hand to make it more comfortable, and I explained that she would soon need to start taking fluids by mouth. However, she was afraid that if she drank, she would have to go to the bathroom a great deal. How could she do this with an intravenous needle in her hand? I told her she would probably use the bedpan at first, but later on in the evening, a nurse would help her get out of bed to use the commode.

LATER POSTOPERATIVE CARE Ms. R. remembered the preoperative teaching well. She coughed and breathed deeply at least every hour or two in the days following surgery, in spite of increased headache whenever she coughed. She did not need to be suctioned. She also did bed exercises and turned herself frequently during her first postoperative day and night.

Ms. R.'s urine output was within normal limits her first operative day. Only once was it considered "borderline excessive," when she voided 300 cc. in a two-hour period. This amount was reported to her doctor, who decided to see what her output would be in the following two hours before ordering pitressin tannate. Her urine averaged 1.000 to 1.015 specific gravity. This was probably due to a slight overhydration more than to a loss of antidiuretic hormone. Her urine was also 2+ to 4+ for sugar and negative acetone, which meant she had to be maintained with regular insulin, in amounts dependent on amounts of sugar and acetone in her urine, throughout the day.

Ms. R.'s postoperative course was considered uneventful by staff members, but not by her. The swelling of her eyelids slowly went down with continued application of the iced compresses, but on her third postoperative day she had an excessive urine output three times in 18 hours. Twice she used the snuffer but the third time she was given a dose of pitressin tannate in oil, intramuscularly. She was upset over the injection, and sure that if she drank less fluid she could control her urine output. We discussed "normal" fluid intake and that no matter how little or how much she drank she would still put out a large amount of urine, for a while at least.

About 10 days after the operation, her helmet was replaced with a stockinette cap. I thought she would see this as a sign of progress, and be happy that only a little of her hair had been removed. Instead, I found her crying. I encouraged her to tell me what she was thinking and feeling.

"I don't know why I'm crying. I just feel like it!"

"Sometimes, after this type of surgery, people do feel like crying and don't know why. It's all right."

"Oh, but it isn't all right at all, nothing's right! I don't feel any better than I did before the operation. I still can't see any better. My urine is still 3+ or 4+, and now I won't be able to have any babies. So, I'm worse off than I was before."

I decided to discuss these specific problems with her. I said it would be three to seven days more before the sugar in her urine would be within "normal" limits, but that many diabetics who have had hypophysectomies experience better control of their hyperglycemia before they leave the hospital. It would be weeks to months before her vision improved, if it did. She might also have to accept the fact that, while it might not improve, at least it probably would not get any worse. I realized, of course, that the latter possibility was not very satisfactory to her at this point. I really did not know what to say about her sterility, other than to agree that sterility is very hard to face. Ms. R., who had said preoperatively that she wanted to have a large family, was thinking about her future as a woman.

When her parents came that afternoon, I told them what the patient had told me that morning. Her parents, her doctor, and I decided she would benefit from counseling with the staff psychologist. However, Ms. R. said that, although she did want to talk about her problems with someone who could help her, she was too embarrassed to talk about sex with a man. She agreed, though, when I explained that the psychologist would treat her the same way her doctor, also a man, treated her and that she could trust the psychologist in the same way she trusted the doctor.

After he had seen Ms. R., the psychologist reported in a team conference that initially she was shy and hesitant, but later opened up to him. He said he believed she was just beginning to go through the second stage in the grief process (developing awareness of loss) over the loss of her child-bearing function. He suggested that we should encourage her to talk about this loss, and to cry whenever she felt like doing so. Her parents, he thought, should have counseling from him and from a gynecologist, so they could help her cope through this stage and the third or restitutional stage which might take several years(10). All agreed that Ms. R. needed to know she could have help whenever she wanted it, and also to have a list of those from whom she could get help.

A week postoperatively. Ms. R. was able to style her short, dark, curly hair so that it covered the scar above her forehead. She measured her urine accurately and consistently. She resumed complete responsibility for testing her urine for sugar and acetone, as well as for giving her own insulin. She was delighted when she realized she had gone for several days with just 1+ or 2+ sugar in the urine. She was tried on 20 units of protamine zinc insulin and 5 units of regular insulin each morning. She responded favorably to this change, and required comparatively little regular insulin otherwise.

Several days before she went home, a program designed to help her control her diabetes was carefully reviewed with her. Diet was the one area in which she needed assistance. She was a slightly built young woman with a fear of becoming fat. The dietitian emphasized that by keeping to a no-concentrated-sweets diet and a good exercise program she would not gain weight.

Before Ms. R. left, I reviewed the hormone replacement therapy with her. Because the hypothalamus would take over the secretion and excretion of antidiuretic hormone, she would probably not have to take this hormone at all, not even on a p.r.n. basis, within a few weeks. She would, however, take home a week's supply of ADH capsules and a snuffer. She would have a prescription for a maintenance dose (25 mg. b.i.d.) of oral cortisone.

Because cortisone therapy can produce muscle wasting and weakness, I suggested that she make sure her diet was high in protein. Also, she had been receiving an antacid with the cortisone, and I suggested that she continue this at home to reduce gastric irritation and the chance of developing a peptic ulcer. We also discussed notifying her doctor if she had an infection or any unusual stress so that he could decide on steroid dosage. She planned to get another card from Medic-Alert, similar to her diabetic card but stating that she was on cortisone and what she needed in case of emergency.

A decision about thyroid replacement was to be made on her first clinic visit. If she showed signs of hypothyroidism, she would be given USP thyroid 15 mg. or sodium levothyroxine (Synthroid) 100 mcg. daily. We reviewed the signs of hypothyroidism which she should report to her doctor at any time.

I also mentioned that she would be given a prescription for a synthetic estrogen, diethylstibestrol 0.5 mg., which she should take each day for 20 days of each month. When she asked, hopefully, if this would possibly restore ovulation, I told her that it would produce menstruation but it would not restore ovulation. The hormone, I explained, would help maintain her normal feminine characteristics. I reminded her that she should report absence of menstruation to her doctor. We agreed it was very important for her parents to know what medications she was taking, and what effects and side-effects they might have on her. Ms. R.'s questions and comments indicated a good knowledge of her medical regimen.

The day she went home, I had many questions myself, questions that only the patient can answer by her life experiences. I knew that she would be returning frequently to the clinic for evaluation of her hormonal status and diabetic condition. She seemed to understand what had been done to her, but I wondered how long she would be able to continue this rather complex hormone replacement therapy. What would she do if her vision did not improve, despite the surgery? What would she do if she had to discuss her sterility with a fiancé? I could only hope that all of us had given Ms. R. and her parents enough support and information to help carry them through life-long therapy. Is the result worth it? This question only time and Ms. R. can answer.

REFERENCES

1. RAY, B. S. Discussion of surgical aspects of pituitary ablation. IN *Symposium on the Treatment of Diabetic Retinopathy* held at Airle House, Warrenton, Va., Sept. 29-Oct. 1, 1968, ed. by M. F. Goldberg and S. L. Fine. (U.S. Public Health Service Publication No. 1890). Washington, D.C., U.S. Government Printing Office, 1969, pp. 422-434.
2. BRADLEY, R. F., AND REES, S. B. Surgical pituitary ablation for diabetic retinopathy. IN *Symposium on the Treatment of Diabetic Retinopathy* held at Airle House, Warrenton, Va., Sept. 29 Oct. 1, 1968, ed. by M. F. Goldberg and S. L. Fine. (U.S. Public Health Service Publication No. 1890) Washington, D.C. U.S. Government Printing Office, 1969, pp. 171-191.
3. DAVIS, M. D., AND OTHERS. Clinical observation concerning the pathogenesis of diabetic retinopathy. IN *Symposium on the Treatment of Diabetic Retinopathy* held at Airle House, Warrenton, Va., Sept. 29-Oct. 1, 1968. ed. by M. F. Goldberg and S. L. Fine. (U.S. Public Health Service Publication No. 1890). Washington, D.C. U.S. Government Printing Office, 1969, pp. 47-53.
4. GUILLEMIN, ROGER, AND BURGUS, ROGER. The hormones of the hypothalamus. *Sci.Amer.* 227:24-33, Nov. 1972.
5. RAY, B. S., AND OTHERS. Pituitary ablation for diabetic retinopathy. Part 1. Results of hypophysectomy (a ten-year evaluation). *JAMA* 203:79-84. Jan. 8, 1968.
6. BELAND, IRENE. *Clinical Nursing: Pathophysiological and Psychosocial Approaches.* 2d ed. New York. Macmillan Co., 1970, pp. 727-728.
7. PEARLSON, O. H., ED. *Hypophysectomy.* Springfield, Ill., Charles C Thomas Publisher, 1957.
8. CHALK, BARBARA. Transphenoidal hypophysectomy. *J. Neurosurg.Nurs.* 3:113-121, Dec. 1971.
9. RAY, B. S. Surgical hypophysectomy in patients with cancer. IN *Hypophysectomy*, ed. by O. H. Pearson, Springfield, Ill., Charles C. Thomas Publisher, 1957, pp. 14-24.
10. CARLSON, C. E., Coordinator. *Behavioral Concepts in Nursing.* Philadelphia, J. B. Lippincott Co., 1970, pp. 102-113.

Cerebellar Stimulation: Pacing the Brain

BRIDGET C. LOETTERLE • MAISIE ROGERS
TINA VALDNER • CARMEN MASON
INA CHRISTIAN • WAYNE ANDREESEN

Uncontrolled seizures and spasticity can incapacitate people with epilepsy, stroke, cerebral palsy, and other brain disorders. This development in functional surgery offers them new hope.

Implantation of a "brain pacemaker" in a patient whose disease is intractable to medications may relieve the symptoms of muscular hypertonia and seizure related to stroke, cerebral palsy, brain injuries, and epilepsy. At St. Barnabas Hospital for Chronic Diseases, New York, New York, 130 such patients have experienced marked functional improvement from cerebellar stimulation. All were nearly incapacitated by their disease.

The cerebellum helps to control skeletal motor activity, but does not produce movement. Rather, the output of the cerebellar cortex is inhibitory, and electrical stimulation of the cortex activates this inhibitory mechanism, which is then directed to deep cerebellar, vestibular, and reticular nuclei cells.

BRIDGET LOETTERLE, *R.N., M.S., was director of in-service nurse education at St. Barnabas Hospital for Chronic Diseases at the time this article was written. She is now assistant professor of nursing, Hostos Community College, Bronx, N.Y.* MAISIE ROGERS, *R.N, is assistant director of nursing at St. Barnabas Hospital for Chronic Diseases.* TINA VALDNER, *R.N., B.S., is head nurse of the neurosurgical unit at St. Barnabas Hospital for Chronic Diseases.* CARMEN MASON, *R.N., and* INA CHRISTIAN, *R.N., are staff nurses on the neurosurgical unit at St. Barnabas Hospital for Chronic Diseases.* WAYNE ANDREESEN *is neurostimulator technician and nursing inservice stimulator instructor at St. Barnabas Hospital for Chronic Diseases. He was the first epileptic patient to receive a cerebellar stimulator.*

Cerebellar stimulation is a non-destructive, functional neurosurgical technique developed by Irving Cooper, M.D., director of the Cooper Institute of Neuroscience at St. Barnabas Hospital for Chronic Diseases, in conjunction with the consulting laboratory. The device consists of a plate of silicone-coated Dacron mesh containing four pairs of platinum-

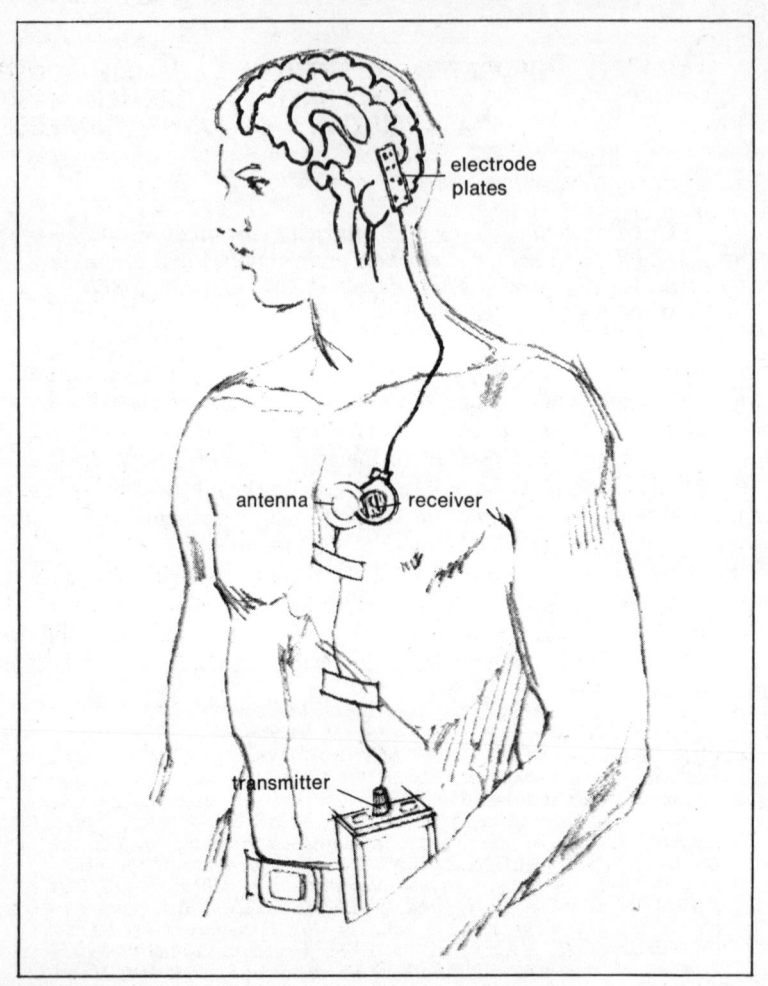

Cerebellar electrodes, *lead wire, and receiver are implanted. External transmitter and antenna provide intermittent stimulation.*

disc electrodes; an internally implanted radio frequency receiver; and a pocket-sized external transmitter.

The electrode plates are applied to the paleocerebellar (anterior) and neocerebellar (posterior) surfaces through small occipital and suboccipital craniectomies. Subcutaneous leads connect the plates to one or two receivers which are implanted in the chest, just below the clavicle, before the brain surgery is begun. Stimulation is controlled by the external transmitter. An antenna is positioned directly over the receiver and the current is delivered through transepidermal inductive coupling.

The electrodes in each plate are stimulated simultaneously in an alternating cycle of several minutes on, several minutes off, so that either the neocerebellum or paleocerebellum is always being stimulated. Rate, frequency, and timing vary with individual patient requirements. The stimulator is fitted with an automatic timer.

Although the criteria for selecting patients have not been defined completely, cerebellar implant surgery is not considered until all other available treatments have been tried. Mental retardation and brain tumor are definite contraindications to implantation; very young children are too immature to cooperate with the procedure.

To date, cerebellar stimulation has not been uniformly successful, but it has enabled many patients to return to normal living or to achieve the coordinated control of movement necessary to further rehabilitation. In patients with seizure disorders, stimulation usually allows a sharp reduction or total discontinuation of anticonvulsant drugs.

No adverse motor, sensory, intellectual, or emotional effects have been noted. Because brain tissue remains intact, cerebral functioning is unaffected. Although it is unlikely that stimulation will alter the natural course of the underlying disease, stimulation may gradually recondition reflex cerebellar function to permit long-term alleviation of symptoms.

Careful evaluation is necessary before surgery. Patients undergo a large battery of neurodiagnostic procedures in addition to routine preoperative tests, including brain scan, cisternography, cerebral blood flow studies, and electroencephalography. A cerebral arteriogram and pneumoencephalogram may be required; for certain spastic disorders, an electromyogram is done. Specialty consultation and evaluation (psychiatric, psychological, speech, pediatric) are obtained if necessary.

Motion pictures are taken of all implantation patients pre- and postoperatively. These movies graphically demonstrate changes due to surgery and provide an accurate, objective tool to evaluate patient status.

Before a patient is selected for cerebellar stimulation, all test results are discussed thoroughly with him and his family. Everyone is given an honest, realistic picture of the situation. In addition to a routine consent form, a special neurosurgical consent is signed. This form clearly details the surgery involved, the stimulation equipment, possible complications, and postoperative routines, and warns the patient that stimulation may not relieve his symptoms.

These patients must remain in the hospital for a long preliminary investigation period and their nursing care is planned to provide safety and psychological support.

Patients with seizure disorders who are on anticonvulsants have frequent determinations of their serum phenobarbital and Dilantin levels. These studies are useful in gauging the therapeutic dose for each patient that will prevent the hazards of toxicity and inadequate dosage.

Most patients with spastic disorders receive dantrolene sodium (Dantrium). Dantrium relaxes muscles by uncoupling the excitation and contraction of skeletal muscle, probably by interfering with the release of activator from the sarcoplasmic reticulum. Dantrium helps control the spasticity associated with stroke, cerebral palsy, and multiple sclerosis. Drowsiness, dizziness, weakness, general malaise, fatigue, and diarrhea are common side effects. The nursing staff constantly observes patients for any of the drug's toxic effects.

Because the preoperative regimen is extensive, the patient and his family need much support. The nurse must establish good rapport and continually supplement the physician's explanations to ensure that everyone understands the purpose of the many diagnostic tests and what to expect during and after the procedures.

The care of children must, of course, include the parents, many of whom have devoted their lives to providing the complex care that chronically ill children need. When introducing and demonstrating the stimulation equipment to a child, the nurse considers his developmental level and modifies her explanations. It is vital that the equipment not be considered a toy.

We are fortunate in having Wayne Andreesen on our staff as a neurostimulator instructor. Wayne underwent the first successful cerebellar-stimulation implantation for intractable, temporal-lobe epilepsy. He visits all potential implantation candidates daily. He counsels them and their families, teaches technical competence in operating the stimulator, acts as a staff resource person, and, above all, is a living example of the positive results that can be achieved. Wayne also works closely with Dr. Cooper and the staff, and is in daily contact with the consultant laboratory to make sure stimulators are working properly and patients are receiving the maximum benefits that can be obtained from them. Tabulation and comparison of current data about each patient provide information that may lead to the design of new and better stimulators.

After a stimulator is implanted, postoperative nursing care is similar to that given any patient undergoing occipital craniectomy. Vital and neurological signs are monitored until they are stable and within normal limits. The patient remains at complete bed rest with his head elevated at a 15- to 30-degree angle for 24 to 48 hours. Bedrest is maintained for five days postoperatively. The occipital and anterior chest wounds are observed to detect infection, drainage, fluid accumulation. or other abnormalities.

Patients with seizure disorders are maintained on at least one anticonvulsant drug to raise the seizure threshold, which may have been lowered by surgery. For five days postoperatively, all patients receive Ampicillin 500 mg. IM every six hours, Decadron 4 mg. IM every six hours, and Talwin 30 mg. IM every four hours for pain.

STIMULATION

Once the patient's condition has stabilized and the operative sites have healed, usually in seven to ten days, stimulation is begun. This is an exciting time for all concerned.

Patients are stimulated at different rates and on varying schedules. Those with seizure disorders usually receive a low rate of stimulation—10 cycles per second—and stimulation alternates every eight minutes between the anterior and posterior cerebellar electrode plates. Patients with spastic disorders ordinarily require a higher rate of stimulation—200 cycles per second—and stimulation is alternated every 16 minutes.

At first, the patient may experience pressure, headache, and a tingling sensation. These symptoms may be more pronounced when higher voltage rates are used. However, these discomforts subside in time, and most patients describe an overall sense of well-being.

When a patient with a seizure disorder experiences the prodromal signs of an attack, he or the nurse should hold the JAM button down until the aura passes, to prevent a seizure. The JAM button is located in the transmitter and activates both antennas so that stimulation occurs simultaneously rather than alternately. The JAM button can also be used to abort a seizure that is in progress.

Most implant recipients remain in the hospital for at least a month postoperatively. During this time the patient and his family are taught how to care for and use the transmitter, and the patient's neurological status is reevaluated by repeating many of the tests done pre-operatively.

The patient's psychological adjustment and his acceptance of this new prosthesis depend greatly on how much improvement and progress he can detect. Therefore, it is vital that he understand that improvement may not be apparent immediately. A long period of stimulation with its cumulative effects may be required to achieve observable progress. For this reason, all of our implant patients are reevaluated within three to six months.

Before he goes home, the patient and his family must be completely familiar with the correct use and care of the stimulator and know how to check to be sure it is functioning properly. Each receives literature prepared by the neurostimulator instructor. Once anxiety is alleviated and the system is understood clearly, the patients realize that the stimulator is really simple to operate.

So far, this still experimental surgery has been most successful in alleviating the functionally incapacitating symptoms of epilepsy and cerebral palsy. The stimulator also has relieved spasticity due to other diseases. Although the long-term success of implant stimulation cannot be determined yet, the marked or complete improvement in function experienced by patients who had limited hope for normal lives is heartening.

Myasthenia Gravis

JOAN STACKHOUSE

Expert nursing care and thorough teaching enable the patient to weather a crisis and cope with this neuromuscular disease.

With gentle, quiet efficiency the nurse moved to suction her patient's tracheostomy, deflate his cuff, and reposition him. Her movements were deliberate and relaxed. He motioned weakly in a prearranged signal and she held a writing slate in place. "Weaker—sudden," he scrawled.

"You're suddenly feeling weaker?" She spoke in calm, measured tones. "All right. We'll be watching you closely and give you what you need." She checked his grip and timed the downward drift of his arms, then moved quickly to the telephone. Moments later the doctor arrived to inject the edrophonium (Tensilon) she had prepared. Immediately the patient opened his eyes and smiled broadly. The dramatic improvement of myasthenia gravis symptoms following the Tensilon test was clearly evident, indicating the patient's need for increased cholinergic medication.

The myasthenia gravis patient requires the highest degree of professional nursing skill. His condition can fluctuate rapidly and with apparent inconsistency. He is usually alert and therefore subject to the emotional trauma of his total dependency and the stress of the ICU environment. The anger, frustration, and fear this patient feels are almost overwhelm-

---

MS. STACKHOUSE, B.S.N., is a public health nurse with the Rockland County Health Department, Pomona, N.Y. She also teaches part-time at Rockland Community College. Ms. Stackhouse prepared this article after caring for a group of myasthenia gravis patients. "However," she writes, "initial interest was thrust upon me in 1954 when I was diagnosed as having myasthenia gravis while I was living in Cameroun, West Africa, and working for the Presbyterian Church." Two years later she underwent a thymectomy which resulted in a complete remission after six years.

ing. His future life style, and his family's, are very much influenced by the quality of teaching and counseling he receives in the hospital.

Myasthenia gravis is a chronic disease characterized by severe weakness and fatigability of various voluntary muscles. It is not a rare disease. Although myasthenia gravis is now diagnosed more frequently, it is estimated that half of all myasthenics are undiagnosed and untreated. Suspecting the disease is still the most important factor in diagnosis. There are an estimated 30,000 cases in the United States. The female to male ratio is six to four. The onset is usually insidious and tends to begin in

---

CLINICAL CLASSIFICATIONS OF MYASTHENIA GRAVIS

Ocular myasthenia
- Involves ocular muscles only (ptosis and diplopia)
- Very mild
- Usually responds poorly to medication
- No mortality; high rate of spontaneous remission

Generalized myasthenia
  Mild
- Slow onset, usually ocular; gradually spreads to bulbar and skeletal muscles but spares respiratory system
- Responds well to medication
- Remission possible
- Low mortality rate

  Moderate
- Gradual onset, usually ocular; progresses to more severe bulbar symptoms and generalized involvement of skeletal muscles
- Responds to medication less satisfactorily
- Restricts activity
- Remission possible
- Low mortality rate

Acute fulminating myasthenia
- Rapid onset of generalized skeletal weakness and severe bulbar symptoms; involves respiratory system early
- Rapid deterioration
- Incidence of crises (myasthenic and cholinergic) frequent
- High mortality rate

Late severe myasthenia
- Severe symptoms develop at least two years after onset of ocular or generalized myasthenia
- Marked bulbar involvement
- Progresses gradually or with sudden deterioration
- Responds poorly to medication
- High mortality rate

Adapted from OSSERMAN, K. E.: *Myasthenia Gravis.* New York, Grune and Stratton, 1968, p. 80.

women between the ages of 15 and 40, and in men over 50, although the disease is also seen in children. Although its etiology is unknown, a defect exists at the neuromuscular junction that causes inadequate transmission of impulses by acetylcholine across the synaptic cleft(1).

Evidence suggests that myasthenia gravis is an autoimmune disorder. Serum antibodies acting against voluntary muscles and certain thymic cells have been identified in myasthenic patients. The high incidence of thymic hyperplasia, the increased number of germinal centers within the thymus, and the fact that thymectomy often produces a remission of symptoms also support the theory that the disease is an autoimmune process. Remissions and exacerbations are characteristic of myasthenia gravis, and it is frequently associated with other diseases thought to be autoimmune, for example, rheumatoid arthritis, lupus erythematosis, and certain thyroid diseases. Infection often causes a worsening of myasthenic symptoms and treatment with immunosuppressives, corticotropin (ACTH), and prednisone is sometimes effective(2).

Approximately one fifth of all myasthenics have ocular myasthenia, and their symptoms do not progress to more serious forms of the disease. Spontaneous remissions are common in this group. On the other hand, these patients often respond poorly to treatment and some must resort to an eye patch to control diplopia.

Persons with generalized myasthenia have some weakness of voluntary muscles and experience various levels of fatigue. Some patients have difficulty walking, climbing stairs, or rising from a chair, but little or no diplopia or severe bulbar symptoms. Others move their limbs with near-normal strength but have such severe bulbar symptoms they can barely talk or swallow. Aspiration and airway occlusion are threats. Respiratory arrest secondary to severe weakness of the diaphragm and intercostal muscles is also possible. The danger of drug toxicity is another hazard, especially in brittle myasthenics. They tend to tolerate only low doses of medication, and, therefore, to go rapidly into either myasthenic or cholinergic crisis(3).

DRUG THERAPY

Cholinergic drugs are the backbone of treatment of myasthenia gravis. With proper medical management, most patients can lead virtually normal lives. The disease was usually fatal until, in 1934, Dr. Mary Walker noted the similarity of myasthenia to curare poisoning and administered physostigmine, the curare antidote, to her myasthenic patient(4). Improvement was dramatic. Since then, analogues of physostigmine, neostigmine bromide (Prostigmin), and pyridostigmine bromide

(Mestinon) have been the drugs of choice in the treatment of myasthenia. Ambenonium chloride (Mytelase) is sometimes used. Drug dosages are carefully manipulated to produce maximum strength with minimal side effects. Most patients prefer Mestinon because fewer side effects. Mytealse is the most toxic of the drugs, but produces maximum strength in some patients.

Cholinergic (anticholinesterase) drugs enhance the effect of acetylcholine at the neuromuscular junction. Normally acetylcholine carries the nerve impulse across the junction to the muscle end plate, and is then destroyed by cholinesterase enzyme. The way is then cleared for transmission of the next nerve impulse. In myasthenia gravis, the impulse is transmitted poorly and becomes progressively weaker. Various theories have been proposed as to the exact location and mechanism of the defect, but the answer is still unknown. However, we do know that inhibiting the action of cholinesterase permits acetylcholine to accumulate in sufficient amounts to transmit impulses more adequately, and that this increases muscle strength. Cholinergic medications do not enable a patient to use his muscles as he did before his illness, but he does become stronger. Enough medication to permit a full return of strength may constitute an overdose, causing extreme weakness and threatening life. The symptoms of over- and underdosage are similar and differentiation is sometimes difficult even for experienced persons.

Tensilon is a valuable tool in diagnosis, dosage adjustment, and differentiation of over- and underdosage. It is effective for less than five minutes. A one cc. syringe is filled using a 10 mg./cc. vial of Tensilon. Initially, 2 mg. are injected intravenously. After several seconds, the patient is evaluated and another 2 mg. are injected. This is repeated until 10 mg. have been given. The patient is evaluated at 30-second, 60-second, and 3-minute intervals.

The patient's baseline strength should be established before Tensilon is given. If he improves, the test is positive and his symptoms are myasthenic. An increase in medication may be indicated. If the patient becomes worse after Tensilon administration, his symptoms are cholinergic and medication is reduced or temporarily withdrawn. A double-blind placebo technique, using saline, is frequently employed to insure validity. Intravenous atropine should be available for use as an antidote when a Tensilon test is performed, in case a severe cholinergic reaction occurs.

Atropine sulfate is used to reduce cholinergic side effects such as gastrointestinal hyperirritability which leads to severe cramps and diarrhea. Atropine dries the secretions stimulated by cholinergic drugs. Some

CHOLINERGIC SYMPTOMS

Symptoms similar to myasthenia:
  difficulty in swallowing
  difficulty in chewing
  difficulty in speaking
  generalized weakness
  difficulty in breathing
  apprehension

Symptoms peculiar to excessive cholinergic therapy:
  abdominal cramps and diarrhea
  nausea and vomiting
  increased, *copious* secretions:
    salivation
    sweating
    lacrimation
    bronchial secretions
  fasciculations
  blurred vision

patients must take atropine daily, but they should be encouraged to take as little as possible since atropine tends to mask the warning signs of impending cholinergic crisis.

Ephedrine is occasionally used to potentiate the actions of cholinergic drugs, and ACTH is sometimes given to patients who have not responded well to cholinergic medication. Usually, 100 units of ACTH are administered daily for 10 days. Since ACTH can cause an initial worsening of myasthenia, it should be administered only in an ICU, where the patient with a tracheostomy has access to a positive pressure respirator. Remissions induced with ACTH usually last from three to six months, so repeated courses are required. Recently, oral, high single-dose prednisone has produced good results in several reported cases. This is still a controversial treatment, but some people predict that prednisone will prove to be the drug of choice in treating myasthenia gravis(5).

THYMECTOMY

In 1939, Dr. Alfred Blalock induced a myasthenic remission by performing a thymectomy, and since then surgery has been an increasingly accepted form of therapy. The best results occur in young women, without thymoma, who have been myasthenic for fewer than five years. However, thymectomy is recommended with greater frequency for men and women up to age 40 who have had the disease more than five years and who are not well controlled on anticholinesterase medication. The thymus is frequently irradiated preoperatively. Results are promising, but remission may not occur until long after thymectomy. A recent study of 267 patients indicated that a remission or improvement was seen in 76 percent of them(6).

The patient should be prepared preoperatively for the possibility that remission may be partial, may not occur for months or years following thymectomy, or may never occur. Since he has depended on cholinergic drugs for months or years, his fears of being off medication during the surgical period must be relieved with careful explanations of how his needs will be anticipated and safeguarded. A system must be devised, with prearranged signals, so that he can communicate his needs, and explanations given that his breathing and swallowing will be eased by a tracheostomy, respirator, and nasogastric tube. If the sternal split incision is to be used, the patient should be prepared for a sternal wound. Low doses of meperidine (Demerol) are usually ordered for pain.

Postoperatively, the patient should be positioned with the aid of a lifting sheet to minimize strain on the incision. A Hemovac or chest tubes may be used. Sterile suctioning technique is important to prevent bronchial and wound infection. Antibiotics are often given prophylactically, and all measures employed to prevent atelectasis and pneumonia. Careful monitoring for myasthenic or cholinergic symptoms is crucial, especially when cholinergic medication is being reintroduced.

Newly diagnosed myasthenics and regulated myasthenics with few symptoms are frequently hospitalized for medication adjustment. Staff should be prepared for the possibility of a crisis. Equipment to manage a respiratory arrest, a spirometer, and intravenous preparations of Tensilon, atropine, and Prostigmin should be readily available.

Either myasthenic or cholinergic crisis can be recognized by the patient's ventilatory distress, difficulty in handling secretions, and severe weakness. He is usually transferred to an ICU. In cholinergic crisis, medications are withdrawn for at least two to three days. Although he is very ill, the patient remains alert and terribly afraid. He needs the support of a calm, competent nurse who constantly reassures him that he will weather this storm, that he will not be left alone. It is very important that he have his own nurse or nurses who care for him consistently.

A baseline of muscular strength must be established and changes closely monitored. Various methods can be used to test the strength of muscle groups, like counting the times the patient can blink his eyelids, raise his arms, or cross his legs; and measuring the degree of ptosis with a ruler. Strength of grips can be measured using a dynometer, or a count made of the times and distances he can pump up the blood pressure machine. Vital capacity should be measured regularly, using the same spirometer each time. What can be swallowed and how many swallows are tolerated should be observed and recorded. Testing is done in relation to the times medication is given. That is, maximum strength can be expected one hour after Mestinon is given, and deteriorating strength three to four hours later. If the opposite occurs, a Tensilon test may determine if the patient's weakness is due to overmedication.

Because infection causes an exacerbation of the disease, the nurse must do everything possible to prevent infection by employing sterile techniques and promoting pulmonary hygiene. A nasogastric tube is usually kept in place to supply fluids and calories. Milk tends to stimulate secretions, and should be avoided when possible. Careful scheduling of care to allow maximum rest should be combined with steps to prevent the hazards of immobility. Special skin care is needed to cope with the diaphoresis and diarrhea which occur with a cholinergic crisis. Constipation should be treated with mild cathartics and suppositories, not enemas, since enemas tend to precipitate a sudden collapse. Weakened eyelids frequently prevent complete closure, and methylcellulose should be used as a conjunctival lubricant to prevent corneal damage.

Of all the stresses confronting these patients in crisis, the inability to speak is the one they mention most often. When they are strong enough to write, a "magic slate" or pen and paper may be used. If his voice is fairly strong and secretions minimal, the patient's tracheostomy may be corked periodically while the cuff is deflated so he can speak. Otherwise the nurse must learn to read lips or arrange a series of signals to be used when the patient is too weak to move. A small hand bell to ring when he cannot call for assistance helps him feel less vulnerable since he can hear it and know that help is being summoned.

PATIENT TEACHING

The patient's need for reassurance cannot be overemphasized. Conversation about the hopeful aspects of myasthenia, and facts about the disease he will want to know when at home are helpful. Above all, the nurse should allow him to express his anger, fears, and frustrations. When the crisis lasts for weeks, as it often does, the patient's despondency deepens. This dependence on the nurse grows and can place a great strain on her.

Patient teaching is done best after he has left the ICU and is again breathing on his own, eating, and speaking. Although he may have expressed a wish to die when he was in crisis, he now dares to believe he will survive and feels it is worth the effort to learn about his illness so that he can manage at home. Things he was told earlier now should be repeated and reinforced. His family must be included in the teaching—and one should not assume that to be told means to be taught. They must know exactly whom to call, where to go, and what to do in an emergency. If the patient is prone to crisis, he should be provided with an Ambu bag and suctioning equipment when he is discharged. He should carry a medical identification card or bracelet.

Patients should learn the difference between myasthenic and cholinergic symptoms, and when and how to take atropine. Unless he is very experienced and stable, a myasthenic should never alter his medication without consulting his doctor. He should be encouraged to lead a normal life, with no activities restricted if he feels able to do them. However, he must maintain a regular schedule, take and record medications exactly as ordered, and eat his meals 30 minutes after taking his medication for optimal chewing and swallowing. Medication taken with a small piece of bread, cracker, or milk may help reduce gastric irritability and nausea. He can avoid excessive fatigue by alternating activities with rest periods, getting a good night's sleep, and pacing himself carefully toward the end of the day. Techniques of self-testing and timing his strength can be introduced. He should be taught to avoid exposure to infection, emotional stress, and activities like frequent stair climbing, that require considerable effort and repetitive movements.

Women should know that menstruation may temporarily worsen their condition, that pregnancy usually is not contraindicated, and that a normal delivery is possible. Some babies born to myasthenic mothers develop a transient neonatal myasthenia in the first few days of life, but it responds readily and permanently to treatment within a few weeks. Young mothers may feel guilty when they are unable to manage all the physical care of their young children. They can be helped to re-order their priorities and to understand that physical care is only one aspect of good mothering.

Many drugs should be avoided or used cautiously by myasthenic patients. These include morphine, ether, quinine, succinylcholine, curare, Innovar, strong cathartics, quinidine, procainamide, steroids (unless given as treatment for myasthenia gravis), and antibiotics which act on the neuromuscular junction, such as streptomycin and neomycin. Sedatives and narcotics should be given in reduced doses when necessary(3). Patients should be cautioned never to take any medication unless prescribed by a doctor who knows them.

Help from every source, hospital and community, should be enlisted —from psychiatry, the chaplaincy, social services, rehabilitation, and others. Many patients benefit from the psychological support and publications of the Myasthenia Gravis Foundation, 230 Park Avenue, N.Y., N.Y., *Help Is On The Way, A Handbook for Patients,* newsletters, and drug bank information.

Most myasthenic patients live full, rich lives despite their disability. Many of them credit much of their success to a particular nurse who nurtured them skillfully and taught them well when they needed help so badly.

REFERENCES

1. MERRITT, H. H. *Textbook of Neurology.* 4th ed. Philadelphia, Lea and Febiger, 1967, p. 549.
2. KINNEY, A. B., AND BLOUNT, M. Systems approach to myasthenia gravis. *Nurs.Clin.NorthAm.* 6:441, Sept. 1971.
3. MYASTHENIA GRAVIS FOUNDATION, NATIONAL MEDICAL ADVISORY BOARD. *Myasthenia Gravis: Manual for the Physician.* New York The Foundation. 1970, pp. 16-17.
4. GREENE, RAYMOND. *Myasthenia Gravis.* Philadelphia, J. B. Lippincott Co., 1969. p. 7.
5. U.S. NATIONAL INSTITUTE OF NEUROLOGICAL DISEASES AND STROKE. *Myasthenia Gravis Research Program.* Washington, D.C., U.S. Government Printing Office, 1971, p. 4.
6. PERLO, V. P., AND OTHERS. The role of thymectomy in the treatment of myasthenia gravis. *Ann.NYAcad.Sci.* 183:308-315, Sept. 15, 1971.

Caring for a Young Addict with Tetanus

CATHERINE M. BOYER

> *The spasms of tetanus had to be controlled if Ms. P. was to survive. When conservative treatment failed, she was curarized.*

Ms. P., 28 years of age, was admitted to the hospital with a diagnosis of possible tetanus. She had a history of drug addiction and of "skin popping" heroin. She was unemployed and had been living with a man who was also an addict.

Tetanus in drug addicts is attributed to two factors: "skin popping" and the use of street heroin which has been "cut" with quinine, a protoplasmic poison. Both provide favorable conditions for the growth of anaerobic organisms. Tetanus in addicts tends to occur more frequently in young, Negro females, and is associated with a more rapid onset of severe symptoms and a higher mortality rate than in non-addict patients(1).

Tetanus is a neurotoxic disease caused by the anaerobic organism, *Clostridium tetani*. The toxin released into the bloodstream by the organism is thought to enter the nervous system, where it is bound at the synapse of the anterior horn cells in the spinal cord, blocking the inhibiting impulses that follow muscle contraction. This causes hypertonicity. The disease process begins at the level of the brain stem and progresses downward. Usually, the first symptom is an inability to close the mouth. The spasms then progress from the large muscles of the back to the extremities(2).

> MS. BOYER *is a graduate of Peter Bent Brigham Hospital School of Nursing, Boston, Mass. and has B.S. and M.Ed. degrees from Teachers College, Columbia University, N.Y. She worked for three years as clinical supervisor of the respiratory intensive care unit at Harlem Hospital, N.Y., and is now director of inservice education at New York Infirmary.*

Nursing the patient with severe tetanus is demanding and challenging. Ms. P.'s care illustrates the complexity of nursing the person with severe tetanus.

On admission, Ms. P. had spasms of her upper back muscles and was unable to open her mouth fully. An initial dose of 5,000 units of tetanus immune globulin (human) was administered; a total of 10,000 units was given over two days to neutralize any circulating toxin. To inhibit the growth of *Clostridium tetani*, a ten-day course of penicillin, 10 million units I.V. daily, was begun. She had an abscess on her left thigh. This was debrided and irrigated with hydrogen peroxide to check this source of continuing toxin release, and a sterile dressing was applied. Our nursing care involved constantly observing Ms. P. for the presence and severity of spasms and any impairment of respiratory function, and providing an environment that was minimally stimulating.

Diazepam (Valium) and morphine sulfate were administered to control the spasms. The use of these medications requires constant observation for diminished respiratory function. Noise and light were reduced as much as possible to minimize the spasms. However, despite medications and other efforts, the severity and frequency of her spasms increased. Ms. P. was conscious at all times—frightened and apprehensive. With each spasm she cried out in pain. We positioned her frequently, as lying flat on her back made her uncomfortable, and remained with her constantly, trying to alleviate her fears by explaining the cause of her symptoms and the purpose of the medications she was receiving.

In the four hours following Ms. P.'s admission, her symptoms became more severe. An emergency tracheostomy was performed to maintain respiratory function, and Ms. P. was placed on a volume respirator. The dosage of morphine was increased and administered hourly. Vital signs were taken every fifteen minutes and a urinary catheter was inserted for accurate output measurement. Phenobarbital (Luminal) was given for sedation. During the next 48 hours, Ms. P.'s condition deteriorated even further. The spasms continued despite frequent, high doses of morphine and Valium. It was decided to curarize her.

Curare (*d*-turbocurarine) is a neuromuscular blocking agent. It acts at the postjunctional membrane of motor nerve end-plate cells where it combines with the cholinoceptive site and blocks the transmitter action of acetylcholine. Normally, a motor nerve impulse results in the release of acetylcholine at the junction, followed by depolarization of the end-plate and eventual muscle contraction. When curare is given intravenously it acts rapidly to cause slight dizziness, a sensation of warmth, difficulty in focusing, and inability to keep the eye lids open. Involvement of the head and neck muscles follows. The limbs become heavy and head movement becomes impossible. Then the ability to move the limbs and trunk is lost. During this time, the patient is conscious and alert. Curare-induced paralysis is brief, but when repeated doses are given, the tissues become saturated and excretion patterns directly influence the intensity and duration of action(3). Curare must be administered at regular intervals to prevent the recurrence of spasms. Because the curare, as well as other medications, must be given I.V., it is imperative that these lines remain patent.

A curarized patient is totally paralyzed. Nursing care is directed at maintaining respiration, muscle tone, elimination, and hygiene; and at preventing infection. Careful attention must be given to the mental state of the patient.

We administered the curare in hourly doses rather than by continuous drip. Ms. P. was given 12 mgs. in 30 ml. of fluid over 15 to 20 minute periods each hour. Once she was completely curarized, it was no longer necessary to minimize external stimuli. During the long period of curarization, we oriented Ms. P. to the time of day and current events, and informed her of all treatments and procedures. External stimulation was provided with the use of a radio. Short periods of undisturbed sleep were allowed between changes of position and vital signs measurements.

Ms. P. remained curarized for 28 days. During this time respiratory function was controlled by a volume-cycled respirator. This respirator delivers a pre-set volume of humidified air mixed with oxygen. All connections from the respirator to the patient must be tight, and any water which collects in the tubing must be removed. The tubing and the distilled water used for humidification are changed and sterilized daily. To determine if the respirator is functioning properly, tidal volumes are measured hourly. An automatic sigh mechanism in the respirator provides complete lung expansion.

Ms. P.'s position was changed hourly, and chest physiotherapy (clapping and vibrating) administered to maintain optimum respiratory function. Following position change and chest physiotherapy, we suctioned her to remove accumulated secretions. Cultures of the tracheal aspirate were taken frequently to detect infection.

The tracheostomy wound dressing was changed every eight hours, and the wound cleansed. The tracheostomy cuff was deflated every hour for one to five minutes depending on Ms. P.'s tolerance. Before the cuff was deflated, the oropharynx was suctioned. Then we used a new sterile catheter to suction the trachea as the cuff was deflated. While the cuff was deflated, we hyperventilated Ms. P. with an Ambu bag connected to oxygen.

We maintained Ms. P.'s skin condition and muscular function with frequent passive range of motion exercises to her extremities and by using a foot board. We frequently changed her position, bathed her often, used skin lubricants and an air mattress, and kept her bed dry and wrinkle free.

Elimination was maintained with enemas. The Foley catheter was irrigated daily with antibiotic solution to minimize the threat of infection.

Nutrition was provided by a continuous drip (36 gtts./min.) of a solution of protein hydrolysate and hypertonic dextrose through a hyperalimentation line in the superior vena cava. We checked her urine every four hours for glucosuria, and when a reaction of 4+ was detected, regular insulin was administered. Sepsis was prevented by the sterile preparation of all solutions and medications, the use of 2 percent iodine at I.V. entry sites, maintaining intact I.V. lines, and the periodic change of the intravenous catheter under sterile conditions.

While she was curarized, Ms. P. was observed constantly. An EKG moniter, with alarms set at 80 and 150, continuously recorded her heart beat, and a simple electroencephalographic recording device monitored brain wave activity during those times when the high doses of medications she was receiving produced unconsciousness. Her pupil reactions were also checked, as curare does not affect this reflex. Blood pressure was recorded every 15 minutes for the first 19 days. Central venous pressure and intake and output were also carefully monitored. During this time Ms. P. also received phenobarbital for sedation and methadone to prevent heroin withdrawal symptoms.

Ms. P.'s course was stormy. The disease process and the many medications made her blood pressure fluctuate continuously. Control of spasms during the first six days of hospitalization was difficult. She developed cardiac arrhythmias and episodes of asystole several times, and required external cardiac massage. During this time she was heavily sedated.

By the beginning of the third week, Ms. P.'s condition began to stabilize. She had periods of wakefulness and sleep. When she was awake, we told her what was happening, why the curare was being used and how it worked, and the purpose of the respirator. Each time we did something for her, we explained what we were doing and why. Since she was unable to communicate with us in any way, we tried to anticipate her needs. The curare dosage was reduced to 7.5 mgs. every hour and no signs of spasm developed. During the fourth week the curare dosage was steadily decreased, and we observed closely for any recurrence of spasm. As the curare dose was tapered, Ms. P. began to communicate with eyelid movement and facial expressions. This gave her a chance to let us know her likes, dislkes, and needs. Later she could write and use her hands.

Her mother visited frequently. Ms. P. had had little contact with her in the past several years, and there appeared to be little warmth or closeness in their relationship. Most of their interactions revolved around resentment and guilt feelings. Her male friend and other friends also visited.

Once the curare was finally discontinued, we began rehabilitation efforts. Our goals included eliminating Ms. P.'s dependence on the respirator through weaning and helping her to regain strength and full muscle function through gradually increased activity and self-care. To wean her from the respirator, we gradually switched it from automatic control to patient control. Then we removed it for ten minutes every hour over a period of days until Ms. P. needed respirator assistance only at night, and then not at all. On her thirty-ninth day in the hospital, her tracheostomy tube was removed. We cleansed the wound and applied a sterile dressing which was changed as needed. The site healed naturally over a few days.

Ms. P. was started on an oral diet beginning with clear fluids and advancing to soft while the tracheostomy tube was still in place. After the tube was removed, she began a regular diet. We encouraged her to help with self-care activities, and she was soon feeding, washing, and moving herself in bed. While she was being weaned from the respirator, we helped her to dangle and then sit in a chair for progressively longer periods. Once Ms. P. no longer needed the respirator, she began walking with assistance.

When Ms. P. left the intensive care area, she continued to recuperate on a medical unit. While she was in the hospital, she was maintained on methadone. Nurses, doctors, and addiction-treatment groups made many efforts to provide drug rehabilitation, but she would have none of this. She refused all help and also was unreceptive to any other teaching efforts. She left the hospital to return to the environment she came from.

Ms. P. was cured of tetanus, a disease with a mortality of about 60 percent. The immunizations she received will protect her from tetanus, but her prognosis in relation to her drug problem is poor.

REFERENCES

1. CHERUBIN, C. E. Epidemiology of tetanus in narcotic addicts. *NY State J.Med.* 70:267-271, Jan. 15, 1970.
2. LAURENCE, D. R., AND WEBSTER, R. A., Pathologic physiology, pharmacology, and therapeutics of tetanus. *Clin.Pharmacol.Ther.* 4:36, Jan.-Feb. 1963.
3. GOODMAN, L. S., AND GILMAN, ALFRED. *Pharmacological Basis of Therapeutics.* 4th ed. New York, Macmillan Co., 1970, p. 608.

Amyotrophic Lateral Sclerosis

MARY A. BOYLE • RUDY L. CIUCA

Complete physical care and sensitive psychological support increase the comfort and significance of life for a patient with this fatal disease.

Mr. A. was a 55-year-old man who was hospitalized with rapidly progressing amyotrophic lateral sclerosis of the pseudobulbar type. He was unable to breathe without a respirator and had difficulty coughing up sputum through his tracheostomy. He was unable to speak or move except to make a few gestures in the air and write with difficulty on a magic slate.

The sounds of the respirator were frightening to Mr. A., who often appeared panicky because of his helplessness. He was tense and depressed much of the time. Although his face was masklike, his eyes spoke eloquently of his despair and suffering.

Mr. A. knew that he would not recover. On several occasions when his respirator was adjusted to provide better ventilation, he made a throat-cutting gesture to indicate that he would rather be dead than go through the agonies of these last ditch mechanical attempts to support his life.

Amyotrophic lateral sclerosis is a fatal disease characterized by progressive degeneration of the anterior horn cells of the spinal cord, the motor nuclei of the lower cranial nerves, and the corticobulbar and corticospinal tracts(1). It usually occurs in persons between the ages of 40

MS. BOYLE, R.N., M.S., is clinical specialist in ambulatory care, Veterans Administration Hospital, Martinez, Calif. She was an instructor at Napa Community College, Napa, Calif., at the time this article was written. MR. CIUCA, R.N., M.S., is assistant chief, Nursing Service, Martinez Veterans Administration Hospital. He previously held a clinical specialist position at this hospital.

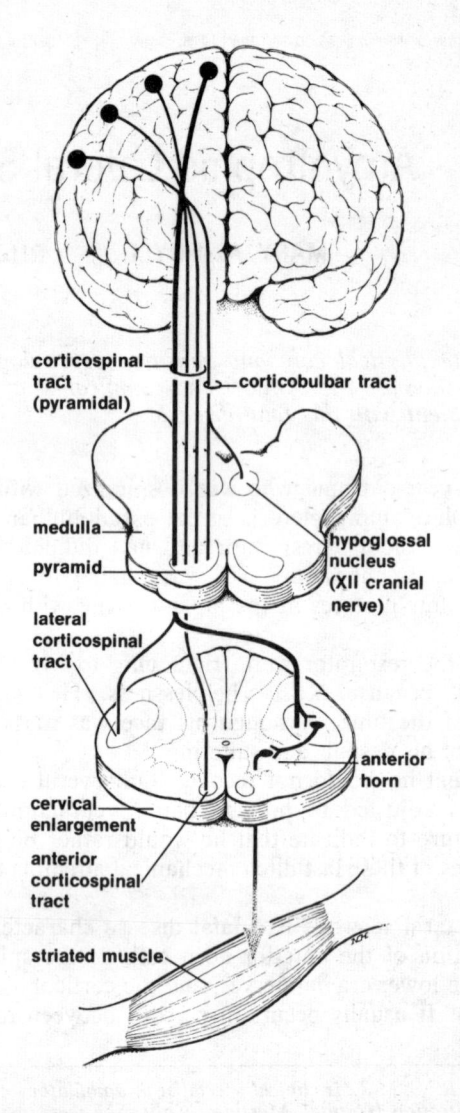

Amyotrophic lateral sclerosis is characterized by degeneration of the pyramidal tract and the motor cells in the anterior gray horns. In cases with corticobulbar involvement the motor nuclei of cranial nerves V, VII, IX, X, XI, and XII also undergo degeneration.

and 70, is more common in men than women, and is of unknown etiology. There is no known treatment.

ALS differs from other motor neuron disorders in its mode of onset, distribution, and progression. ALS is characterized by steadily progressive muscular weakness, cramps, fasciculations (which are almost always present), and wasting.

In poliomyelitis, on the other hand, muscular fasciculations and fibrillations decrease as strength increases. In multiple sclerosis, they may appear and disappear with remissions and exacerbations. Some neuropathies begin more abruptly than ALS, progress to a plateau, then go into remission. Nerve conduction patterns usually are abnormal in other motor neuron diseases, but in ALS they are normal in the presence of marked muscle atrophy(2).

Weakness and fasciculations may appear in any muscle or group of muscles. The upper limbs may be affected first, most commonly with wasting and weakness of the intrinsic muscles of the hands. A Babinski reflex is present and tendon reflexes are hyperactive. (Babinski reflex refers to the dorsiflexion of the foot and large toe with fanning and abduction of the other toes and flexion of the knee and hip.)

If the symptoms appear first in the lower limbs, they usually are more noticeable on one side and the patient says that his legs feel tired and heavy(3).

When ALS is of the bulbar type it interferes with the hypoglossal, spinal accessory, vagus, and trigeminal nerves. Eye movement is not impaired. There are fasciculations of the tongue with increasing loss of articulation, facial expression, and ability to chew and swallow. The tongue may be weak and atrophied.

Slurring of speech is due to spasticity of the tongue and lips. Respiratory muscles weaken, leading to dyspnea and shortness of breath. Eventually death is caused by aspiration, pneumonia, and respiratory failure. Loss of sphincter control is rare: if present, it occurs late in the disease. There are no paresthesias or apparent sensory changes: the person's mind remains alert until death.

On the average, patients live about four years, but those whose ALS commences with bulbar palsy may die within a year(4). Patients without bulbar involvement may live as long as nine years.

NURSING CARE

Nursing care for Mr. A. consisted of physical support, prevention of complications, and psychological comfort and support as he went through the terminal stages of illness.

His physiological needs were those of the totally dependent person who requires outside intervention to meet the simplest, most basic daily needs. Physical care had a definite psychological impact and vice versa. Therefore, nursing management was directed to Mr. A. as a unified whole. Support of his remaining adaptive mechanisms, both physiological and psychological, was of the utmost importance to avoid adding further stressors to his already taxed state.

Nursing intervention, Byrne and Thompson point out, is less than effective if nurses divide stress into separate entities, such as psychological and biological stress, when the patients resultant state is, in fact, singular and he can only be observed and treated as a unified whole(5).

In planning care for Mr. A., we considered the nature of the stressors he was coping with. Before his illness Mr. A. had worked, played, socialized with friends, and lived in a lovely home with his wife. A few months later he was in a hospital bed with no control over his environment, no ability to participate in any activities. He could not eat, drink, or talk, and could not breathe without the respirator. Nursing care was aimed at assisting him to make the most appropriate use of his remaining energy.

Central to Mr. A.'s care was the establishment of a trust relationship between him and his caretakers, a relationship based on the recognition that Mr. A.'s illness was catastrophic and terminal, that he was still working through the grief process and probably was still in the anger phase, and that he was completely dependent physically.

Mr. A.'s depression was obvious, as were his nonverbal expressions of helplessness and hopelessness. With certain stimuli he would cry openly with grief and loss. At other times his attitude was one of sorrow at his impending loss of everything and everybody.

It was important that Mr. A. know that we wanted to communicate with him and satisfy his needs. We responded to his feelings and wishes with promptness and understanding. When he made his throat-cutting gestures, for example, we avoided false reassurances, held his hand, and let him know that we realized he was in a desperate situation.

Receiving get-well cards was difficult for Mr. A. He seemed to appreciate these messages, but after he read them he always cried, then became depressed. Since he did not want us to talk about his feelings, we held him by the hand, let him see our sadness and tears, and quietly remained with him until he was able to gather his resources.

Because Mr. A. feared the respirator and was distressed at his helplessness, we spent as much time with him as possible, to show him that he was still a valuable person, that we were concerned, that he would not be rejected, and that he would be cared for in any emergency.

When Mr. A. was alone for even an hour, he became increasingly restless and put on his call light about every 10 minutes. His pulse rate increased, his pupils dilated, and he hyperventilated, over-riding the respirator, and thus making his breathing more labored. As his breathing became more difficult, his anxiety would increase. This pattern would continue until he became exhausted. He usually required increased doses of Valium (diazepam). This was particularly noticeable on the evening and night shifts when there were fewer people around.

Before we understood what was happening we had thought of Mr. A. as a demanding patient. For example, we had difficulty getting out of his room because he always thought of one more thing for us to do right away.

The night nurse stated that the respirator often became dislodged from the tracheostomy and she wondered if Mr. A. did this as a death attempt. However, because the apnea alarm sounded whenever the respirator was off the tracheostomy, we soon realized that this was Mr. A.'s one sure way to get someone to come into his room. As we spent more time with him, this behavior ended and he became considerably less restless and tense. His fears and needs were anticipated before he made the demand.

Increased contact with Mr. A. gave us an opportunity to become skilled at interpreting his nonverbal communication. This was important because, if the communication was too complicated or the nurse was not tuned in, he became frustrated and exhausted. Hence, anticipating the meaning of Mr. A.'s nonverbal communication was a main point in the nursing care plan.

Our communication was even more essential because Mr. A. had very few visitors and those that did come stayed only a few moments, unable to cope with his helplessness and their own fright. Mr. A. sensed this and was often depressed after his visitors left.

Toward the end of his illness he had no visitors except his wife, who came in for a few minutes once a day. A very reserved person, Ms. A. did not discuss her feelings with the staff despite our attempts to draw her out. She stated that she knew his illness was terminal and that he would not live much longer. She seemed composed and accepting of the whole situation. Like her husband, she was reluctant to discuss it, so we did not try to force communication.

Because Mr. A. was unable to take any part in his personal hygiene, we tried to involve him in decisions about it. He had a heavy "five o'clock shadow," and we learned that he had always shaved twice a day. Asked if he wanted this continued in the hospital, he said yes, and we shaved him during his morning and afternoon care.

Keeping Mr. A.'s airway patent and supporting his respirations was a major nursing responsibility. Because Mr. A. had difficulty coughing up sputum, his tracheostomy was particularly worrisome to him. He was reluctant to have a student nurse suction his tracheostomy until an instructor had gone through the procedure step by step.

Since he could not tolerate being off the respirator for more than the few moments it took for suctioning, the instructor took that opportunity to explain to both Mr. A. and the student the method, technique, and significance of suctioning. She demonstrated, then had the student return the demonstration. Throughout, Mr. A. was asked his opinion: Was he comfortable? Did the tube feel clear? Could he breathe adequately? When he responded in the affirmative, his conclusions were reinforced.

Later Mr. A. conveyed to the student that no one had ever explained the proceudre to him before and now that he understood it he was comfortable allowing her to suction him. It also helped him feel more secure if the nursing staff checked his tracheostomy and respirator frequently. His tracheostomy was cleansed three times daily and suctioned as necessary.

Mr. A.'s muscles were so weak that he was unable to sit in a chair. His sternocleidomastoid muscles would not support his head and his shoulder girdle was too weak to support his arms and upper body. Therefore, he was bed bound, and because he could not tolerate lying flat due to his weak respiratory muscles, he usually lay in semi-Fowler's position.

We turned him every two hours from side to back to side. Although Mr. A. did not have strength to turn himself, he could grasp the side rails, so we encouraged him to do this as it gave him a sense of participation. At this time his skin was carefully inspected for redness and pressure areas, and lotion was applied to the bony prominences. Mr. A. was on an alternating pressure mattress. Trochanter rolls were used to prevent outward rotation of his legs, and a bed cradle to keep the bedclothes off his legs and feet.

He was given a complete bath every day with particular attention to his back and perineum, and range of motion exercises to all his limbs four times a day. This helped maintain muscle strength and ease his frequent leg cramps. We explained the physical care procedures and solicited his opinions regarding the degree of comfort they afforded.

Mr. A. was given oral hygiene twice daily with a toothbrush and paste. Since he could not swallow, a suction machine and tonsil tip were also used. Lemon-and-glycerin swabs and mouthwash were employed throughout the day for mouth comfort.

Fluids and nutrition, administered by nasogastric tube, were major items in Mr. A.'s nursing care. A total of 3,000 cc. of fluid were given daily, about one third consisting of Sustical and the rest of water. These feedings had to be given hourly since a larger amount at one time produced gastric distention and impaired his respiratory function. We arrived at this schedule through consultation with Mr. A., who was able to indicate when the feeding was too much and made him uncomfortable and when it was a tolerable amount.

Because he had entered the hospital in a dehydrated, malnourished state, it was essential to improve his nutritional status to the best possible extent, and to help prevent urinary tract infection by providing adequate fluids. He also needed to be observed for gastric and abdominal distention since the semi-Fowler's position is not conducive to optimal gastric and intestinal motility.

Mr. A.'s bowel movements were regular and his urinary output was adequate. His intake and output were measured, however, because patients in his condition are prone to constipation, impactions, and decreased urinary output.

Mr. A. slept only for 30 to 45 minutes at intervals throughout the day and night, so it seemed best to group his activities around his sleep periods. As much as possible, he was suctioned, turned, and given his tube feeding at one time.

We found that Mr. A. was very bright and enjoyed watching news programs. This provided him with some outside stimuli. His care was arranged so that he would have the energy to watch these programs. We scrupulously avoided communication between each other that did not include Mr. A. This required some effort since there is a tendency to "talk about" the person who cannot speak, forgetting that he can hear and understand very well.

Although Mr. A. seemed to enjoy our attempts to amuse him, we were careful in using this approach lest he get the impression that he was surrounded by people who didn't understand the seriousness of his predicament.

Throughout our relationship there was a certain sadness and feeling of futility because Mr. A.'s physical condition was deteriorating and our ability to intervene in the process was negligible. It seemed important to help him find some meaning in his situation by providing the best nursing care we were able to give and including him in the decisions about his care. We hope this made it easier to accept the things that had to be done for him and gave him some sense of control and participation. Perhaps our frequent visits and efforts to communicate told him of our concern and our desire to provide comfort and support as he faced his catastrophic illness.

Mr. A.'s respiratory status continued to deteriorate. Soon he was too weak to use the Bird respirator. He died of respiratory arrest eight weeks after his admission to the hospital, 18 months from the onset of his first symptom.

REFERENCES
1. ELLIOTT, F. A. *Clinical Neurology*. Philadelphia, W. B. Saunders Co., 1971, p. 242.
2. KENRICK, M. M., AND SUSKIEWICZ, LEWIS. Review of suspected cases of amyotophic lateral sclerosis *South.Med.J.* 65:707-710, June 1972.
3. MERRITT, H. H., ED. *A Textbook of Neurology*. 5th ed. Philadelphia, Lea and Febiger, 1973.
4. ELLIOTT, *op.cit.*, p. 245.
5. BYRNE, M. L., AND THOMPSON, L. F. *Key Concepts in Nursing*, St. Louis, C. V. Mosby Co., 1972, p. 48.

Section IV Traumatic Neurological Damage: Acute Care and Rehabilitation

The articles in this section deal with the devastating effects—both immediate and long-term—of traumatic injury to the central nervous system. The acute care of persons who have sustained craniocerebral trauma is the focus of the first two articles presented here. Early detection of brain damage and intervention to reverse its effects can minimize morbidity and prevent death. The remaining articles deal with the measures nurses can take to help the patient who has sustained central nervous system trauma to attain the optimum level of function possible for him—physically, emotionally, and mentally.

Craniocerebral Trauma

ANN HINKHOUSE

The patient with a head injury has possibly sustained permanent damage to his central nervous system. Nurses can do much to prevent further morbidity by observing the patient for early signs of a change in his condition.

The cranium is a relatively closed, rigid vault, containing the brain, cerebrospinal fluid, and blood. Its total contents must remain approximately the same at all times. If there is a change in the proportional volume of any one of these components, the others must compensate for the change. A progressive increase in the volume of one component results in increased intracranial pressure with accompanying neurological symptoms(1).

Craniocerebral trauma involves injuries ranging from a jarring of the nerve cells, with minimal histological changes, to fractures and hemorrhages. The degree of increased intracranial pressure and interruption of nerve cell structure and function which a patient experiences varies directly with the severity of the injury.

A minor injury with minimal pathology (concussion) generally produces only a temporary loss of consciousness, but may cause minute hemorrhages. This bleeding usually causes only a minor increase in intracranial pressure.

Subdural and epidural hematomas are usually associated with a significant head injury. An epidural (extradural) hematoma usually results

MS. HINKHOUSE is a graduate of Lutheran Hospital School for Nurses, Moline, Illinois, and holds a B.A. degree from Cornel College, Mt. Vernon, Iowa. She is a nurse clinician and evening supervisor on a surgical nursing service at the University of Iowa Hospitals and Clinics, Iowa City, Iowa.

from a severe head injury associated with a skull fracture and a tear in the middle meningeal artery. The hematoma forms between the dura and the skull causing rapid compression of the brain since the hemorrhage is arterial. Subdural hematomas are usually caused by lacerations of the veins crossing the subdural space. Because of the venous origin of the bleed, symptoms may develop slowly. Hemorrhages may occur with or without fractures.

Linear skull fractures usually are not surgical emergencies because they involve a change in bone continuity without distortion. Comminuted fractures are multiple linear fractures with fragmentation of the bone. If these fragments are displaced, the fracture is called depressed. A skull fracture with bone protruding through an external opening—the scalp, mucous membranes, or eardrum—is a compound fracture. Fractures are frequently associated with injury to the underlying brain substance.

In assessing the patient with craniocerebral trauma, the emergency room nurse must determine the level of injury with which she is dealing. She should attempt to learn from the patient or from witnesses and ambulance attendants how, when, and where the injury was sustained; whether there was loss of consciousness, and its nature; the position and movement of the patient after the injury; whether there was vomiting and its nature; and any pupillary changes.

Knowing how the injury was sustained helps one anticipate what changes may occur in the patient's condition. For example, if a traumatic injury resulted from penetration of a sharp object, as in a gunshot wound, there is a greater chance of intracranial infection than if the patient fell against a blunt object and sustained a closed head injury.

In addition to the risk of infection, intracranial hematomas from this type of injury can be rapidly fatal. Foreign material and bone fragments must be removed unless critically situated. Irrigations with antibiotic solutions are vital. Signs of trauma are more visible in the open injury, but the nurse should observe for signs and symptoms of slow subdural bleeding in a closed injury. If head trauma occurred secondary to seizure or syncope, this information is useful in anticipating future episodes of unconsciousness.

The patterns of loss of consciousness which occurred before the patient arrived at the hospital are also significant. For example, an epidural hematoma can be suspected if the patient experienced the classical pattern: immediate loss of consciousness, followed by a lucid interval, and then by a progressively stuporous state. In a subdural hematoma, the patient experiences a lucid interval followed by a gradual loss of consciousness. Any history of unconsciousness warrants observation of the patient for a period of time after the accident.

If the patient exhibits decerebrate posturing, the nurse can anticipate life-threatening problems, such as respiratory distress, due to the possible brainstem damage associated with a cerebral injury severe enough to produce this posture. If the patient is flaccid, one considers not only cerebral damage, but possible neck injury, and takes steps in turning or positioning him to protect against further spinal cord damage.

Vomiting is not uncommon after trauma due to the emotional and physiological impact of the situation. Projectile vomiting, however, can indicate increased intracranial pressure. Similarly, pupillary dilatation and inequality may indicate increased pressure and also help identify the cerebral hemisphere involved. Changes in pupil size and reactivity provide valuable information if changes are recorded over a period of time. Therefore, any observations made by ambulance attendants should be included in the patient's record.

The patient is observed for a varying length of time, depending on the severity of the injury. If he experienced only a momentary loss of consciousness, has negative skull x-rays and no positive neurological findings he may be discharged after a brief period of observation. An excellent opportunity for health teaching is available since some neurological symptoms do not appear for hours. The patient and his family can be given a written check list of important signs (such as nausea, vomiting, pupillary changes, lethargy, drowsiness, or difficulty in being aroused from a sleeping state) which, if they develop, indicate a need to see a physician. The emotional stress associated with an injury may cause friends and relatives to forget these symptoms if only verbal instructions are given. A patient who might develop symptoms is occasionally admitted to a temporary observation unit associated with the emergency room.

In addition to observing and noting the patient's initial condition, the emergency room nurse frequently must begin life-saving care for the severly injured patient.

There are many unknown factors in caring for the head injury victim. If the patient arrives in an unconscious state, the nurse must consider the possibility that other conditions exist. Is the patient postictal or hypoglycemic? Has he ingested nonprescribed drugs or failed to take prescribed drugs? Is he inebriated? Is he having an hysterical reaction? Falls resulting in head injury may be associated with any of these conditions, and information from witnesses may be helpful in pin-pointing the cause of the injury.

After the nurse completes an initial assessment of the patient and assures his adequate ventilation and circulation, she must establish an

EARLY MANAGEMENT OF THE PATIENT WITH CRANIOCEREBRAL TRAUMA

Problem	Action
Inadequate airway	Position head with jaw jutting outward to prevent tracheal obstruction—do not move neck Remove foreign materials from mouth, including dentures Check for oral bleeding Insert airway to keep tongue forward Intubate and give respiratory assistance if positioning does not restore breathing Observe for chest trauma Prepare equipment to draw arterial blood specimen
Vomiting	If necessary, turn patient to side keeping spine in alignment with head, to prevent aspiration Have suction available for immediate use Insert nasogastric tube
Circulatory collapse	Apply pressure dressings to actively bleeding areas Draw blood for CBC and type and crossmatch Start I.V. of balanced electrolyte solution (e.g. lactated Ringers), especially in presence of multiple trauma; flow rate 100 cc./hr. Check blood pressure and pulse q 10-15 min Insert indwelling urinary catheter Observe for abdominal and thoracic injuries DO NOT place in Trendelenburg position
Level of consciousness	Note precise LOC when patient arrives If patient is fully alert, obtain information from him regarding his accident Observe for progressive drowsiness and irritability If unconscious, record nature and degree of response to mild and painful stimuli
Seizure	Maintain airway Do not restrain patient, but protect him from falling or otherwise injuring himself Record starting point, parts of body involved, duration Note deviation of eyes, if any
Condition of pupils	Observe size, quality, reaction to light, deviation from midline Check q 15 min for bilateral or unilateral changes, especially dilatation Remove contact lenses if present
Drainage of blood or cerebrospinal fluid from nose or ears	Apply sterile, loose, dry dressing Note quantity, consistency, and color of drainage
Scalp lacerations	In active bleeding, apply pressure dressing If not bleeding, irrigate well with sterile normal saline; wash area, shave in preparation for suturing

individualized plan of care. This includes recording vital and neurological signs, observing changes in the patient's level of consciousness, checking for associated injuries, and arranging for diagnostic procedures and admission to an inpatient area.

A change in the level of consciousness is the single most important factor in the observation of a patient with a head injury. The patient's orientation deteriorates first to time, then to place, and last to name (2). A patient who has regained consciousness in the emergency department must be continually observed for the development of progressive stupor. This change occurs earlier in the progression of an injury than do focal neurological signs(3).

Depending on hospital policy, the patient with craniocerebral trauma may spend less than an hour or several hours in the emergency department. Therefore, secondary assessment may begin there or in an in-patient unit. This assessment includes changes in the patient's neurological status and level of consciousness as well as late-developing symptoms of head and other bodily injuries.

Initially, the blood pressure may be within normal range. If intracranial pressure rises, blood pressure rises as a reflex response to cerebral anoxia, affecting the vasomotor cells. The pulse may vary at first and then slow as the blood pressure rises. Respirations may be labored at first and eventually become intermittent as increasing intracranial pressure leads to anoxia of the respiratory center in the medulla(4). The patient's temperature signifies little about increased intracranial pressure but should be taken after the patient's first evaluation since fever increases the metabolic needs of an already deprived brain(5). Except for severe brainstem injuries, febrile states are not likely to result from cranial injuries.

The third cranial or oculomotor nerve regulates many of the changes in the pupils. Increased pressure on this nerve causes ipsilateral (same side) dilatation. On direct stimulation with light, there is a progressive slowing of pupillary contraction and eventual fixation. When performing this test, one uses a flashlight with a strong and concentrated beam and examines each pupil individually. If the corpus callosum between the two cerebral hemispheres is intact, there will be a simultaneous consensual reaction of the unstimulated pupil even though there may be no reaction to direct stimulation. Some people normally have unequal pupils(6).

The position and movement of the patient's extremities can indicate other neurological deficits. Is abnormal posturing present? Is it continuous or intermittent? Are the patient's hand grips equal and strong? Is movement restricted on one side of the body or in all extremities? Are there signs of decerebrate posturing with rigid extension of all extremities, abduction of the arms, arching of the back, and toes pointed inward? Or is there decorticate posturing in which the patient's arms are abducted in rigid flexion and the hands are rotated internally? Is the patient's response to stimulation purposeful? Decreased movement and sensation may be related to spinal cord injury, but motor fibers passing downward from the midbrain can be compressed cranially, producing symptoms similar to those seen in cord injuries(5).

Maintaining a quiet environment can help alleviate the restlessness commonly associated with increased intracranial pressure. Emergency rooms are frequently noisy. If possible, head-injured patients should be isolated from noisy patients. The patient with craniocerebral trauma occasionally speaks in loud and abusive tones, but the nurse should avoid talking loudly to the patient. Answering his questions in a simple, direct manner helps to minimize his confusion. The patient should also be protected from having bright lights shine directly on his face. Elevating his head at a 15 degree angle, unless contraindicated by circulatory collapse, often keeps him quieter and more comfortable. This position also helps reduce cerebral edema. The nurse must check for other conditions which might cause agitation, such as bladder and bowel distention, poor oxygenation, and pain.

Depending on the nature of his head injury, the patient may be restless enough to require restraint. If possible no more than two or three extremities should be restrained. Leather restraints are generally the best since they are strong and safe. Strips of gauze bandage can be looped around an extremity which has been padded with a folded washcloth. With any restraint, observe the foot or hand for distal edema. Padding the side rails of the cart or bed with bath blankets helps to protect the patient against further injury. Unless contraindicated by an intracranial hematoma, the nurse can place the patient on his side to make him more comfortable as well as to prevent aspiration of oral secretions and prolonged pressure leading to decubiti.

An accurate intake-output record is important. The person with a moderate to severe craniocerebral injury usually has an I.V. started for the administration of medications and to maintain adequate hydration. Overhydration must be avoided since increased intracellular volume increases cerebral edema.

The nurse must explain the basic aspects of the patient's care to his relatives and friends, in addition to answering their questions about his level of consciousness and degree of orientation. They are aware that the patient may have permanent, partial, or total loss of control over his phys-

MEDICATIONS AND FLUIDS USED IN THE EMERGENCY TREATMENT OF HEAD INJURY

Medication	Usual Dose	Route	Action
Dexamethasone (Decadron)	6-10 mg. initially; 4-6 mg. q 4-6 h	I.V.; IM	Rapid acting glucocorticoid; acts on glial cells and neurons to prevent or reduce cerebral edema. (Questionable efficacy in trauma, but given for possible benefit.)
Glycerin 10%	1-1.5 Gm/kg. over 24 hours	I.V.; po	Osmotic diuretic for reducing cerebral edema.
Mannitol 18%	250-500 cc. over 8 hours	I.V.	Osmotic diuretic; draws fluids from extracellular spaces to reduce cerebral edema.
Diazepam (Valium)	5-10 mg. initially; repeat q 30 min. p.r.n.	I.V.	Acts on hypothalamus and thalamus to terminate or reduce seizure activity.
Diphenylhydantoin (Dilantin)	50-100 mg. q 8 h	IM; po	Acts on cerebral cortex as anticonvulsant; usually requires 24-48 hours to reach effective levels.
Phenobarbital (Luminal)	30-60 mg. q 8 h	IM	Depresses motor cortex to prevent or terminate seizure activity; infrequently used in acute head trauma due to depression of sensorium.
Ampicillin (Polycillin)	1-2 Gm. q 6 h	I.V.; IM	Broad spectrum antibiotic. (Antibiotics are used sparingly in the first 24 hours following injury, except in basilar skull fractures with otorrhea or rhinorrhea.)
Tetanus toxoid	0.5 cc.	IM	For passive immunity in presence of cranial trauma. (May require two subsequent booster doses at 4-6 week intervals if not previously immunized.)
Human Tetanus Immune Globulin	250-500 units	IM	For active immunity in cases of severely contaminated cranial wounds.
Codeine	30 mg.	IM; po	Analgesic. (Narcotics are usually avoided in head trauma due to generalized CNS depression.)
Acetaminophen (Tylenol)	325-650 mg. q 4 h p.r.n.	po; pr	Analgesic
Acetylsalicylic acid (Aspirin)	300-600 mg. q 4 h p.r.n.	po; pr	Analgesic
Propoxyphene (Darvon)	32-65 mg. q 4 h p.r.n.	po	Analgesic
Dextrose 5% in Water with 30 mEq. NaCl/liter	40-60 cc./h	I.V.	To provide some calories without large quantities of electrolytes. (Adrenal response to trauma causes electrolyte retention.)
Normal Saline (0.9%)	cc./cc of gastric drainage from nasogastric tube q 8 h	I.V.	Maintenance of electrolyte balance by providing exact replacement of output. (No added K due to increased serum K level from tissue breakdown in trauma.)

Basic principle in I.V. therapy in craniocerebral trauma: dehydration of patient to reduce extracellular fluid volume which causes cerebral edema.

ical and social activities as a result of the injury, and are justifiably worried about his prognosis. It is advisable to avoid the word comatose in describing the patient since this word has a multitude of meanings to the public. Instead, stating that the patient is not speaking at present gives concrete information without requiring the nurse to define vague terms or make predictions.

The patient's history and his condition on arrival in the emergency room provide valuable baseline information for those who will care for him in the future. Since she is often responsible for the care of the head-injured patient for the first few hours after injury, the professional nurse in the emergency room has opportunities to use observation skills as well as techniques of emergency care.

REFERENCES
1. GIUS, J. A. *Fundamentals of General Surgery*. Chicago, Year Book Publishers, 1957, p. 652.
2. QUESENBURY, J. H., AND LEMBRIGHT, PAMELA. Observations and care for patients with head injuries. *Nurs.Clin.North Am.* 4:239, June 1969.
3. HAY, RANKIN. Head injuries. IN *Emergency Room Journal Articles,* ed. by Abraham Gelperin and Eve Gelperin. Flushing, N.Y., Medical Examination Publishing Co., 1970, p. 210.
4. YOUNG, J. F. Recognition, significance, and recording of the signs of increased intracranial pressure. *Nurs.Clin.North Am.* 4:225, June 1969.
5. QUESENBURY AND LEMBRIGHT, *op.cit.,* p. 241.
6. *Ibid*, p. 226.

Respiratory Changes in Head Injury

L. CLAIRE PARSONS

Hyperventilation, hypoventilation, and impaired cellular respiration can rapidly contribute to the development of secondary brain injury—some of which is preventable.

During the past 50 years, more deaths have occurred in the United States from traffic accidents than the total number of lives lost during the Revolutionary War, the War of 1812, the war between the states, the numerous disputes with the Indians and Mexicans, the First and Second World Wars, and the Korean conflict(1). Every year, 100,000 persons die from trauma in this country. In the under-44 age group, it is the leading cause of death. More than half of trauma fatalities are due to highway accidents and, in over 70 percent of this group, head injury is the prime cause of death(2).

Complicating the pathophysiologic sequelae of head injury in the trauma patient is the increasing frequency of alcohol and drug-alcohol intoxication(3). The official United States statistics, from 1955 to the present, indicate that 25 percent of automobile accidents are related to alcohol intoxication; this does not include the 25 to 30 percent of the people involved in accidents who refuse to permit a blood analysis for alcohol content(4). Further complicating the evaluation and treatment of the accident victim is the widespread occurrence of drug abuse. Thus, the head-injured patient may arrive in the emergency room as a neuro-

---

DR. PARSONS *received her B.S. in nursing from Northwestern State College in Natchitoches, La.; her M.S. in biology from the University of Houston, and her Ph.D. in physiology from the University of Texas Medical Branch in Galveston. Dr. Parsons holds a joint appointment in the University of Virginia School of Nursing and School of Medicine.*

physiologic enigma with his central nervous system possibly traumatized by mechanical, chemical, and pharmacologic abuse. Even if a complete evaluation of the neurologic status of such a patient is not possible, there are usually changes in vital functions which, if immediately corrected, can control or possibly prevent further neurologic deterioration.

To understand why rapid and competent care is so important, let us digress for a moment and consider the mechanisms responsible for cerebral damage in head injury. Head trauma may be grouped into two general categories; open head trauma and closed head trauma.

OPEN HEAD TRAUMA Open head trauma results from a sharp instrument or projectile penetrating the skull and disrupting the underlying dura mater, leptomeninges, and brain tissue. Cerebral lesions caused by sharp instruments tend to be localized, permitting the resulting cerebral dysfunction to be predicted with more accuracy than in closed head injury.

CLOSED HEAD TRAUMA Closed head injuries result from sudden acceleration or deceleration of the head and present a rather different clinical picture. Cerebral lesions that result from closed head injury may present a wide variety of neurologic signs and symptoms, which make it difficult to evaluate or predict the extent of damage. Spatz classifies such injuries as primary and secondary according to their origin(5).

Primary lesions are those that are due to the mechanical disruption of cerebral tissue at the time of impact(6). They may be focal or multifocal in character. Morphological changes following the primary cerebral tissue damage in closed head injury include contusions of the soft membranes and cerebral cortex, primary medullary hemorrhages, and epidural, subdural, and subarachnoid hemorrhages(7).

Secondary brain lesions are generally accepted to be the result of circulatory dysfunction and post-traumatic cerebral edema(8). These complicating factors can cause partial or total necrosis of cerebral tissue, ischemic nerve cell changes, and diapedetic hemorrhages in which corpuscular elements pass through intact vessel walls into brain tissue(9).

While the physician-nurse team has no control over primary lesions inflicted by initial brain trauma, experimental evidence suggests that secondary lesions, caused by circulatory impairment and cerebral edema, may be minimized by expert care immediately following the trauma.

PRIMARY BRAIN TRAUMA: RESPIRATORY CHANGES

Even before a nurse touches a patient with head injury, she may observe respiratory abnormalities. A review of the effects of head trauma on respiratory function provides several useful nursing principles which can guide the practitioner who is giving care to the patient with a head injury.

HYPOVENTILATION Some investigators indicate that, when flat or hyporespiration is observed in an unconscious, head-injured patient who has simultaneous injury of the facial bones and cranium, frequently the patient has an upper airway obstruction due to an accumulation of blood and mucus in both the nasopharyngeal space and trachea(10). Establishing a clear airway with an adequate supply of oxygen can have a tremendous effect on the prognosis. In fact, MacIver and other investigators have shown that measures improving airway-lung function and oxygenation decrease the mortality in head-injured patients from 90 to 40 percent(11). Tracheostomy, when indicated, decreases the mortality from head injury by 10 to 15 percent(12,13).

If the patient arrives in the emergency unit in a hypoventilating state, the ultimate outcome will depend on whether he has suffered reversible cerebral concussion or more extensive brain damage which has resulted in either cerebral contusions or intracranial hemorrhage. Some investigators believe that, in a concussion, the respiratory changes are due to pulmonary rather than brain dysfunction; with more extensive brain damage, respiratory changes indicate primary brain dysfunction(14). In either case, ventilation must be assisted when hypoventilation exists in the head-injured patient.

In a relatively short time, hypoventilation produces respiratory acidosis. Carbon dioxide accumulates in both blood and lungs, while the oxygen content of these compartments decreases (see diagram, page 142).

The increase of carbon dioxide in the blood to the brain dilates the cerebral blood vessels, which increases cerebral blood flow. The increase in blood supply and in the amount of oxygen released at the tissue level due to decreased pH represents a compensatory mechanism on the part of the patient to maintain an adequate supply of oxygen and nutrients to the vital cerebral tissues. If hypoventilation continues beyond the compensatory state, cerebral hypoxia and edema will damage the brain parenchyma, imposing a secondary brain trauma.

HYPERVENTILATION In the severely head-injured patient, hyperventilation and respiratory alkalosis may occur. Despite an increased minute volume, oxygen desaturation can develop in the tissues. These changes in respiration can be due to aspiration and atelectasis immediately after

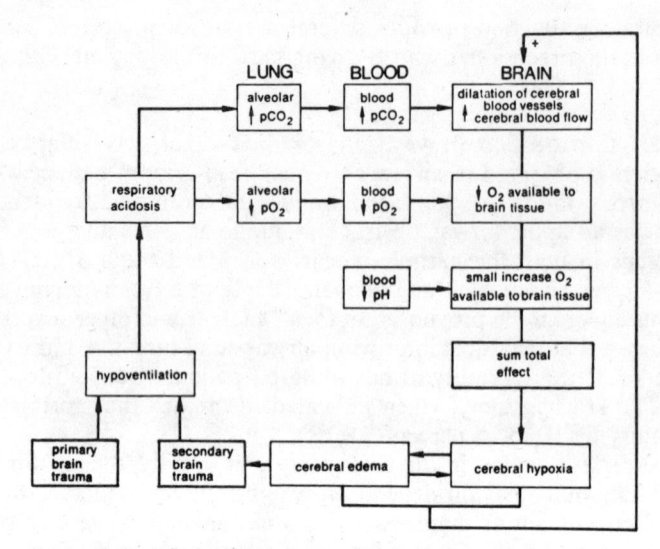

Hypoventilation following brain trauma results in respiratory acidosis. As the carbon dioxide increases and the oxygen decreases in the blood and lungs, cerebral hypoxia and edema produce secondary brain trauma.

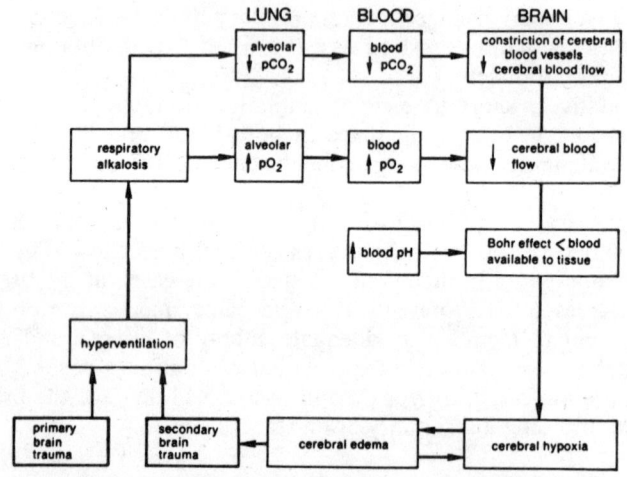

Hyperventilation following brain trauma produces respiratory alkalosis. Although the oxygen in the blood and lungs increases, the decrease in carbon dioxide causes constriction of the cerebral blood vessels and, as in hypoventilation, secondary brain trauma results.

head injury(15). They may be related to lesions in the pons(16). Or they may possibly constitute a compensatory response to cerebral edema(17).

If unchecked, hyperventilation will develop into respiratory alkalosis. The decrease in the carbon dioxide content of the blood reaching the brain tends to constrict the cerebral vasculature, decreasing cerebral blood flow. The decrease in blood supply and the subsequent decrease of oxygen released at the tissue level due to vasoconstriction may result in cerebral ischemia and hypoxia despite the increase in oxygen in the blood (see diagram, this page). Impaired cerebral blood flow due to cerebrovascular spasm and cellular disruption of brain tissue may further compromise the function of the injured brain.

SECONDARY BRAIN TRAUMA:
CIRCULATORY DYSFUNCTION AND CEREBRAL EDEMA

Research conducted by several investigators reveals that hypoxia of the brain, resulting from acute closed craniocerebral trauma, leads to

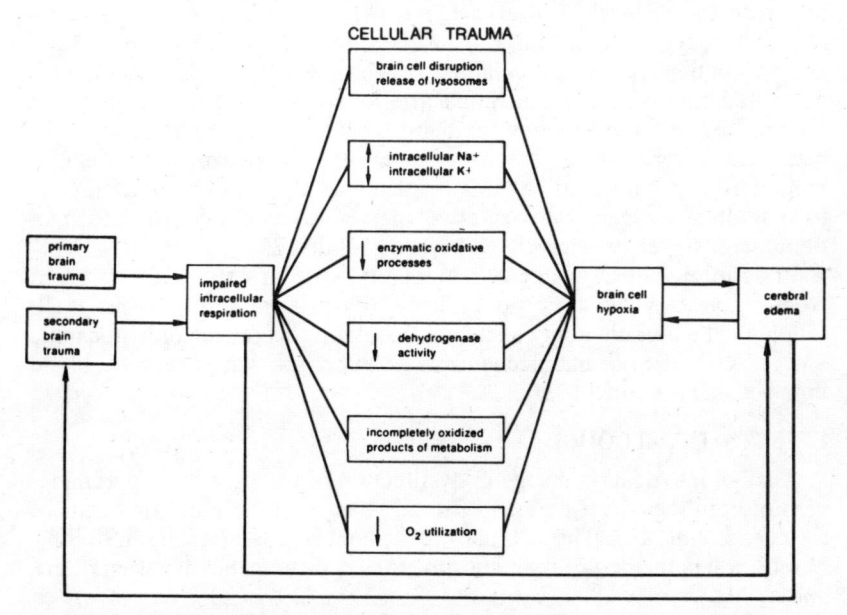

On the cellular level, the effects of primary and secondary trauma impair intracellular respiration. This results in a variety of cellular dysfunctions which produce brain cell hypoxia, cerebral edema, and further secondary brain trauma.

depression of the enzymatic-oxidative processes and accumulation of incompletely oxidized products of protein, carbohydrate, and lipid metabolism cerebral tissue (see diagram, page 145).

The dehydrogenase activity and oxygen utilization of the brain tissue drops to 40 to 50 percent of its normal level, and brain hypoxia and cerebral edema ensue(18,19).

In a study of the arterial and venous cerebral blood gases of 27 patients immediately following severe craniocerebral injuries and brain surgery, Forwein and other investigators found that, in the surviving injured patients, the arterial pO_2 was diminished from the normal 95 to 100 mm.Hg to a mean of 76 mm.Hg, while the venous pO_2 levels remained within normal limits or only moderately decreased. The head injured patients with a fatal course were found to have a mean pO_2 of 64 mm.Hg and severe venous hypoxia.

Leibzon and Kozyrev reported similar findings in 20 patients with severe craniocerebral trauma accompanied by prolonged loss of consciousness and disturbances of vital functions. They also found that, within 24 hours following a severe head trauma, venous cerebral blood pO_2 rose to the level of arterial blood pO_2(20). Thus, the large arteriovenous oxygen level difference, seen initially in Forwein's "fatal course" patients, can be explained on the basis of blood stasis and a decreased rate of perfusion. Small arteriovenous (A-V) differences, as seen in Leibzon and Kozyrev's patients 24 hours after trauma, may indicate that cerebrovascular spasm or massive impairment of cellular metabolism or both exist. At this point, the brain tissue becomes unable to assimilate oxygen, the oxidative metabolic processes are nonfunctional, and severe cerebral tissue hypoxia results(21).

In addition to pO_2 changes, patients in Forwein's study also suffered from respiratory alkalosis, as indicated by arterial pCO_2 levels of 30 mm.Hg. The investigators concluded that, with this degree of hypocapnia (low pCO_2), the normal mechanisms of autoregulation of cerebral blood flow become nonfunctional(22).

EFFECTS OF ALCOHOL

Alcohol intoxication results in dysfunction of ganglion cells, pyramidal cells of both the motor area and frontal lobes, and the Purkinje's cells of the cerebellum(23). This cellular impairment results in abolition of inhibitions, a lengthening of reaction time, and a discrepancy between desire and ability.

When experimental guinea pigs were given ethyl alcohol intraperitoneally and subsequently concussed, there was a significant delay in the onset of cerebral edema. This may have been due to the diuretic effect of

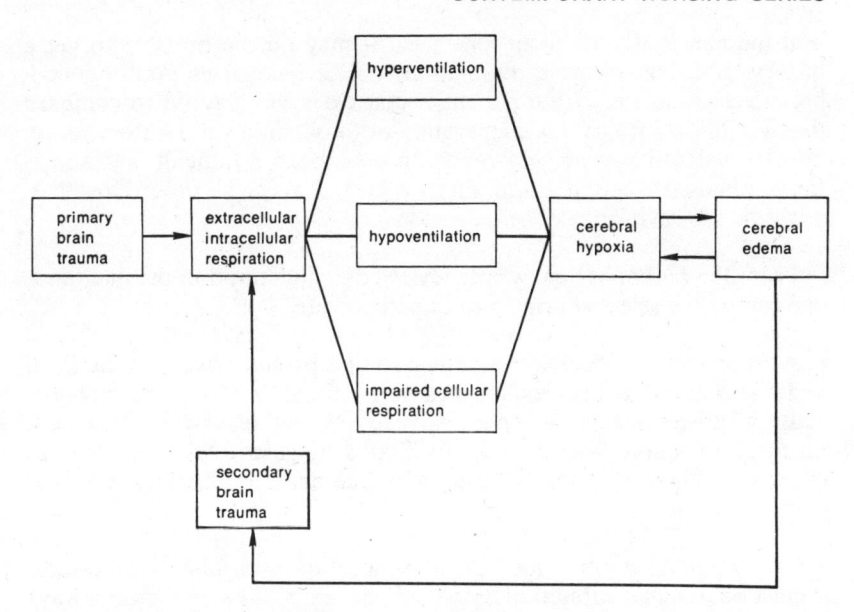

```
                    ┌──────────────────┐
                    │ hyperventilation │
                    └──────────────────┘
┌─────────┐   ┌──────────────┐   ┌───────────────┐   ┌──────────┐   ┌──────────┐
│ primary │   │ extracellular│   │               │   │ cerebral │   │ cerebral │
│ brain   │──▶│ intracellular│──▶│ hypoventilation│──▶│ hypoxia  │◀─▶│ edema    │
│ trauma  │   │ respiration  │   │               │   │          │   │          │
└─────────┘   └──────────────┘   └───────────────┘   └──────────┘   └──────────┘
                    ▲            ┌───────────────────┐
                    │            │ impaired cellular │
                    │            │ respiration       │
                    │            └───────────────────┘
              ┌───────────┐
              │ secondary │
              │ brain     │
              │ trauma    │
              └───────────┘
```

Initial brain trauma *generally results in respiratory changes noted by hyperventilation, hypoventilation, or signs of impaired cellular respiration. Without intervention, secondary brain trauma ensues and a cycle of increasing cerebral damage develops.*

alcohol, which tends to inhibit the antidiuretic hormone (ADH). Cerebral edema developed about two hours later and persisted for a significantly longer period than the cerebral edema in experimental concussion without alcohol(24).

In an uncontrolled patient situation, when a traumatic brain injury is superimposed on the alcoholically depressed brain, the prognosis becomes poor because of the difficulty in trying to evaluate the patient's condition: a decreased level of consciousness may be due to brain trauma or inebriation. Vomiting and bradycardia may be due either to increased intracranial pressure or to alcoholic intoxication. Also, the "pseudo-protective" diuretic effect of alcohol delays the formation of cerebral edema until the alcohol has been metabolized. Trying to manage the cerebral edema which finally occurs after alcohol has been metabolized is more difficult because, when it does develop, it persists for a longer period of time than cerebral edema without alcohol ingestion(25). In addition, if an inebriated head-injured patient is brought into the emergency room unconscious, it may not be possible to get a history, and signs of brain trauma may not be recognized until the alcohol effects wear off. If the patient is conscious, he may be so confused that it is difficult to get his cooperation or to obtain a valid history. Also, his physical and psychologic condition may make it difficult, and sometimes impossible, to perform diagnostic and surgical procedures that might be life-saving.

From the pathophysiology just reviewed and pictured in the diagrams, one can derive selected principles of patient care.

PATENT AIRWAY Never leave a patient until a patent airway is functional and respiration has been established at a normal rate and tidal volume. Take whatever means are necessary to prevent aspiration of blood, mucus, or vomitus. This may be facilitated by gastric lavage as well as removal of blood and mucus from the mouth and throat with gentle oropharyngeal suction.

ASSISTED VENTILATION If mechanical support of respiration is necessary, it must be initiated without delay. A mechanical respirator should always be available for use and in good repair. Several tracheostomy trays or setups as well as mechanical suctioning equipment are absolutely necessary.

FLUID RESTRICTION Both oral and parenteral fluids should be restricted. Do not routinely start intravenous fluids without restricting the flow to minimal rates, because of the impending danger of cerebral edema.

LEVEL OF CONSCIOUSNESS Try to ascertain the level of consciousness as soon as possible. It is important to determine how the patient answers questions—coherently, incoherently, or not at all—and how he responds to mechanical stimulation, beginning with a light touch and progressing to deep pain.

If the patient is coherent, try to obtain information about his last meal, alcohol or other drug consumption, hypersensitivities, and any history of metabolic diseases (as diabetes mellitus) or neurologic deficits. It is very helpful in evaluating the patient to find out if he remembers the accident, the events preceding and subsequent to the trauma, and if he has remained conscious since the head injury.

An audiomagnetic tape recorder is a useful tool in obtaining and temporarily storing information. A patient's answers can be recorded and used in evaluating his level of consciousness immediately following trauma, as well as several hours later. The recording of this kind of information may also prove useful in differentiating between speech associated with alcohol or drug intoxication and that due to traumatic lesions of the brain.

EYE REACTION In checking the patient's eyes one must evaluate both pupillary reaction and eye movement. Each pupil must be checked to determine if it is constricted or dilated, and how it responds to light—sluggishly, rapidly, or not at all; the two pupils are compared to each other to determine if they are equal in size and reaction to light. If nystagmus is present, the direction—horizontal, vertical, or rotary—should be noted.

RHINORRHEA OR OTORRHEA Determine if the patient is having drainage from the nose or ears and note the color, consistency, and amount.

VITAL SIGNS Frequent checks of vital signs, such as heart rate and blood pressure, are obviously cardinal in caring for the head-injured patient. Bradycardia, increased blood pressure, and restlessness are signs suggesting neurologic deterioration.

A patient with a head injury, particularly a closed head injury, may enter the emergency room as an enigma. The signs and symptoms of brain injury may be masked or potentiated by alcohol or other drugs; the head trauma may not be obvious and there may be no one to relate a history of head trauma; and the patient may or may not be conscious or coherent enough to relate his own history of head trauma. However, if the patient exhibits any signs of possible head trauma—contused or lacerated head, impaired ventilation, increase or decrease in blood pressure and pulse, decreased level of consciousness, nose or ear drainage—he should be evaluated and when necessary treated for brain injury. Otherwise, secondary brain injury may rapidly ensue and irreversible damage may occur.

REFERENCES
1. CAMPBELL, H. E. Deceleration and the motor car. *JAMA* 154:1023, Mar. 20, 1954.
2. NATIONAL ADVISORY NEUROLOGICAL DISEASES AND STROKE, COUNCIL SUBCOMMITTEE ON HEAD INJURY. *Survey of Current*

Head Injury Research; a report. Bethesda, Md., National Institute of Neurological Diseases and Stroke, 1969.
3. LANDAUER, A. A., AND OTHERS. Alcohol and amitriptyline effects on skills related to driving behavior. *Science* 163:1467-1468. Mar. 28, 1969.
4. IMIELINSKI, L., AND LIPINSKA, D. Alcoholic intoxication as a factor complicating actue cranio-cerebral injury, *Wiad.Lek* 20:1991-1966, Nov. 15, 1967.
5. SPATZ, H. Pathologische Antomie mit besonderer Brucksichtingung der Rinderkontusion. *Zbl.Neurol.Psychiat.* 78:615-616, 1963.
6. *Ibid.*
7. UNTERHARNSCHEIDT, F., AND SELLIER, K. Pathomorphologie der gedeckten Schadelhirn verletzunger. IN *Proceedings of the Third International Congress of Neurological Surgery,* held at Copenhagen. Aug. 1965, edited by A. C. de Vet and others. New York, Excerpta Medica, 1965, pp. 63-73.
8. SPATZ, *op. cit.*
9. UNTERHARNSCHEIDT, T. AND SELLIER, K. *op. cit.*
10. KURTZ, T., AND PITTS, F. W. Management of closed head injuries. *Surg.Clin.Am.* 48:1271-1278, Dec. 1968.
11. MACIVER, I. N., AND OTHERS. The role of respiratory insufficiency in the mortality of severe head injuries. *Lancet* 1:390-393. Feb. 22, 1958.
12. ULIN, A. W., AND ROSOMOFF, H. L. Management of airway in acute head injury. *Arch.Surg.* 67:756-761, Nov. 1953.
13. DUNSMORE, R. H. AND OTHERS. Tracheostomy in neurosurgery. *J.Neurosurg.* 10:228-232, May 1953
14. GRUBB, R. L., AND OTHERS. Respiration and the cerebrospinal fluid in experimental cerebral concussion. *J.Neurosurg.* 32:320-329, March, 1970.
15. FROMAN, C. Alterations of respiratory function in patients with severe head injuries. *Br.J.J.Anaesth.* 40:354-360. May 1968.
16. PLUM, F., AND SWANSON, A. G. Central neurogenic hyperventilation in man. *Arch.Neurol.Psychiat.* 81:535-549, May 1959.
17. LUNDBERG, N., AND OTHERS. Reduction of increased intracranial pressure by hyperventilation. *Acta Psychiat.Neurol.Scand.* 34 (Suppl. 139): 5-57. 1959.
18. FROWEIN, R. A., AND OTHERS. Is there sufficient oxygen supply in the brain tissue following severe brain trauma? *Zbl.Neurochir.* 25:39-60. 1964.
19. GOTOH, F., AND OTHERS. Cerebral effects of hyperventilation in man. *Arch.Neurol.* 12:410-423, Apr. 1965.
20. LEIBZON, N. D., KOZYREV, V. A. Saturation of the arterial and venous blood with oxygen in acute closed craniocerebral trauma (experimental and clinical investigation). *Vop.Neirokhir.* 28:8-12, May-June 1963.
21. SCHMIDT, C. F. Twenty years of cerebral blood flow measurements. *Cir.Res.* 11:357-359, Sept. 1962.
22. FROWEIN *et als., opt. cit.*
23. HOFF, H. *Lehrbuch der Psychiatrie.* Wien, Bruder Hollinek, 1956.
24. MUSIL, F. Influence of ethyl alcohol on the course of brain edema after injuries. *Rozhl.Chir.* 44:753-759, Nov. 1965.
25. IMIELINSKI, L., AND LIPINSKA, D. *op. cit.*

Nursing Rehabilitation After Severe Head Trauma

EDITH NORSWORTHY

Brain injury causes cognitive and intellectual deficits which not only hamper the patient's sensory and motor functions, but also may destroy his sense of self.

If you've ever awakened away from home and not known where you were; if you've traveled in a foreign country and didn't know the language; if you've tried to do Christmas shopping with a cast on your leg; if you've struggled to make a cake, only to have it fall; then you may have an inkling of what it's like when your "I-ness" is scrambled because of a head injury.

Care after a head injury is helping a person put himself back together so he can function in his environment. This kind of caring takes time, flexibility, and sensitivity.

The true challenge in nursing the brain-damaged patient is to create an environment where the patient's established methods of attending to his physical disabilities also serve to treat the intellectual, cognitive disabilities that accompany severe head injury. A nurse does not "take care of" a patient striving for rehabilitation; she plans her assistance so that the sum total of her interventions and the patient's abilities equals accomplishment. And she gears her therapy to increase the patient's level so that her assistance can diminish. The nurse is a therapist, and the goal of her therapy is to enable her patient to deal with his environment. She

---

MS. NORSWORTHY *(BS.N., Medical College of Georgia, Augusta; M.S., Boston University, Boston, Mass.) was a nursing care consultant at Rancho Los Amigos Hospital, Downey, Calif., at the time this article was written.*

works to minimize his limitations, and to enhance his adaptive capacities, and his ability to be himself in spite of his limitations.

Weakened or lost muscular control and impaired speech are the more obvious, predictable symptoms of brain injury. Less easily recognized but perhaps more devastating, if they are not taken into account during the patient's rehabilitation program, are the behavioral changes that result from central nervous system damage. Interference with intellectual functioning, decreased ability to make decisions, and lowered capacity for self-responsibility are usually concomitant symptoms that must be recognized and dealt with throughout treatment.

One can view the patient's recovery as moving along a continuum. At the outset are the simple, egocentric, directed-by-others, dependent activities. At the other end are the more abstract, complex, sociocentric, self-directed, and independent accomplishments. It is vital that those responsible for his care be sensitive to where the patient is on this continuum, and that the demands put on him are commensurate with his capabilities at that given point. Structuring his activities so that he is aware of his achievements gives the patient a feeling of success and a sense of personal worth. Push him too fast, so that he fails to meet expectations—yours and his—and you only impede his progress. Therapy should reinforce his successes at each stage of his rehabilitation, and create opportunities for him to progress to the next level.

PATHOPHYSIOLOGY

Knowing the function of the various parts of the brain is helpful in relating trauma to symptomatology. The frontal lobe of the cerebrum is responsible for the initiation, organization, and inhibition of volitional activity. It mediates personality, the "I" concept, and self-direction in judgment. Injury to the frontal lobe results in decreased affect, a flat, unemotional personality. The person so injured may have marked difficulty in beginning, maintaining, or ending a task. For example, a hungry man may stop feeding himself for no apparent reason, or he may continue bringing the fork from the plate to his mouth long after his food is gone.

Together, the parietal, temporal, and occipital lobes receive information, compare it with previous knowledge, and attach meaning to it. Input to the parietal lobe comes through the skin, pressure, temperature, and position senses of body parts. This information is used to discriminate the size, shape, and consistency of tangible objects. A parietal lobe dysfunction leaves sharp-dull sensation intact, but the individual cannot gather information by his sense of touch. In other words, he must gather information in other ways than through touch.

The temporal lobe receives auditory information, compares it with previous input, and attaches meaning to it. Dysfunction of the temporal lobe results in a receptive aphasia; the person cannot understand what he hears. Therefore, he may mimic what he hears or appear to totally disregard it. He may break into jargon because he is unable to monitor his speech; in effect, he cannot hear himself speak.

HOW TO PROMOTE SELF-FEEDING

PROCEDURE: Minimal distraction feeding (MDF)

PREREQUISITE:
1. Taking oral diet.
2. Able to feed self at least portion of meal independently.

PURPOSE: To limit distraction so that the person's attention is more likely to be maintained on eating. The environment is modified to compensate for the person's disability.

NOTE: MDF is NOT used to isolate a messy eater who is objectionable to others. If the current priority goal for the individual patient is socialization, MDF is used judiciously.

INDICATIONS: Evidence of impaired attention:
1. Stops eating before food is gone
2. Leaves the eating situation before finished
3. Unable to socialize and eat simultaneously
4. Reaches for other objects in the eating setting.

ESSENTIAL STEPS	KEY POINTS
A. Procedure 1. Place person alone with reduced visual stimuli (curtains drawn, or facing away from activities). 2. Keep food and utensils to a minimum. Place only salad and fork on tray. When salad is finished, place plate with meat and fork on tray. 3. Increase number of foods given at one time as the person progresses. 4. Move to dining room, but seat at own table. B. Recording 1. When therapy is instituted, write nursing order and enter on Kardex under problem and approaches. 2. Evaluate effectiveness at patient-centered conferences and note in the progress notes.	A patient who is overstimulated at mealtime mixes all foods with his fingers, throws food and utensils, and is generally agitated and displays other 'brain-damaged' behaviors. Drugs are often given for these. However, a therapy organized around a daily event can reduce agitated behavior and raise the level of independence.

Visual information is received through the occipital lobe, compared to previously received information, and given significance. Complete loss of occipital lobe function causes "cortical blindness"—sight is no longer a functional sense. Damage to the occipital lobe impairs one's ability to receive cues from what one sees.

The functions of the parietal, temporal, and occipital lobes, which comprise the posterior cerebrum, are interrelated, and cues received from each lobe aid in the associative processes of them all. The common, integrated, or gnostic area correlates information from the three lobes, educing conclusions that are unavailable to any individual lobe. Impairment of the gnostic area inhibits reaction to sensory cues, even though the three lobes may be intact.

In summary, then, the posterior cerebrum makes decisions based on the information it receives. These decisions are relayed to the anterior cerebrum, which initiates the desired activity. The motor strip, located in the frontal lobe, directs voluntary movements. The brain and brain stem are pathways that relay messages from the body and its receptors to the brain, and relay directions from the brain to the body. Disorders of movement, such as tremors, rigidity, and dystonia, result from damage to the midbrain, pons, and medulla. The cerebellum is another mediating pathway of motor activities. Coordination, balance, posture, and rhythm are impaired when the cerebellum is damaged.

An understanding of these overlapping, interrelated brain functions helps explain why good physical care is only a part of what the patient needs. Physical care influences the other symptomatology. How a patient is given food and water, how he receives treatment to prevent hazards of immobility and compensate for lost body function affect not only his primary disorder, head trauma, but also his efforts to orient and organize himself.

Comprehensive care of the brain-damaged patient also requires an understanding of the physiological basis for his behavioral inconsistencies. Thereafter, assessment of his abilities and disabilities is an ongoing process. Performance must be measured day-to-day so that emerging patterns can be predicted and treated. Just as no two people respond identically to a situation, so, too, each brain-damaged patient's behavior differs as he interacts with his environment. To be effective, treatment must be specific. This requires a careful evaluation of each area of interaction with his environment that the patient finds difficult. The relationship of a disability to the specific damaged area can be deduced from observed behavior. Behavior can be broken down into components which readily suggest intervention. Because it is the person's behavior that is ultimately seen and judged by society, behavior is the focus of much of rehabilitation.

DISRUPTION OF INPUT

Following a severe head injury, one major problem is the impairment of certain sensory receptors. Because decision making and subsequent behavior rely on information received through the individual's data collecting senses, a breakdown of this system at the input stage can lead to maladaptive behavior.

What can be done to augment the patient's information gathering faculties? During the period of coma, when the patient does not respond to verbal stimuli, egocentric information can be supplied in various ways. Without observable responses, we can only assume reception of our input. This means we do not talk *about* the patient within his hearing, but we do talk to him.

As he becomes more alert, the patient tends to turn toward noises, to focus his eyes on objects, and to attend visually if these objects move. Although his five senses are now more responsive to input, the person is not selective in his attention. At this point, intervention should be directed toward structuring situations to aid the patient in selection. We can begin to give him basic training in attaching meaning to input. Extraneous stimuli should be eliminated. One would not, for example, attempt activities-of-daily-living training in a group setting at this stage of rehabilitation. Words, touch, and gestures are used to focus the patient's attention on the directions that are given.

Besides difficulty with selection, the person has a limited attention span. Therefore, he should not be kept at one task or asked to maintain his attention on one stimulus for an extended period. Indeed, an attempt to push him beyond this limit increases error and frustration, which discourage his effort. For example, when assisting the patient to assume self-feeding, we can divide the task into units of activity interspersed with periods of rest.

Tactile sensation and proprioception, also components of a person's information-gathering equipment, may be deranged or absent, making it necessary for him to rely more heavily on any visual cues which are involved. Hemianopsia, other visual field deficits, and diplopia are common. Attention to the placement of the patient's bed and selection of his place at the dining table are methods of encouraging compensation for his deficits, as is reminding him to look to see if his fingers are near the spokes of the wheel chair.

Not all sensory receptors are impaired in all patients, or in equal

HOW TO PROMOTE URINARY CONTINENCE

PROCEDURE: Bladder training for male patient when incontinence is due to low level of consciousness or impaired cognition.

PREREQUISITE: Urological management until patient has low residual urine and indwelling catheter has been removed.

PURPOSE: To establish controlled voiding for increased self-esteem and social acceptance.

ESSENTIAL STEPS	KEY POINTS
A. Procedure 1. Help patient focus attention on elimination. Be nonjudgmental: "You are wet" or "You need changing."	(a) This is egocentric information, given to compensate for impaired selectivity of attention. (b) Must be aware of differences between wet and dry, clean and dirty, before he can proceed to Step 2. (c) Previously, patient has not had to think about controlling elimination.
2. When patient can communicate his awareness of need to be changed, begin to focus on anticipation. Continue to be nonjudgmental: "Did you realize you were going?" or "Can you feel it when you urinate?"	This communication of awareness is often nonverbal (restlessness, looking around —presumably for the bathroom). It can be effective communication only when staff members are consistent, observant, and skilled in interpreting these observations.
NOTE: At this stage the patient may be inconsistent in communicating his need. His awareness of the need to urinate may come too late to prevent accidents. To remove the external catheter at this point and push for continence usually leads to failure.	Staff members can be more patient and supportive of a person who has a low frustration tolerance if they themselves experience success and have definite guidance with therapeutic approaches.
3. Leave external catheter in place, but ask the patient to indicate when he needs to void. At 'usual' voiding times, such as on arising and after meals, the staff should ask the patient "Have you voided?" or "Do you feel the need to void?"	Involve the entire team at this point in order to develop and reinforce more consistent communication of anticipation. Attention and memory are both necessary to succeed at this and all following steps. He must be able to remember your instructions and attend to the task at hand and attend to bodily sensations.

ESSENTIAL STEPS	KEY POINTS
Reinforce these questions by either (a) disconnecting the catheter from the leg bag and allowing voiding through the catheter into the urinal, or (b) simply examining leg bag to see if there is urine there.	This should continue to be a low-pressure procedure. Recognition of success is usually reinforcement enough, but gold stars on a chart have been particularly rewarding to some patients.
4. After three or four days of consistent successes at Step 3, remove the external catheter. Continue to suggest toileting to patient.	The patient needs success, and he needs to be rewarded for it. Continue the reminders. Arrange his clothing and receptacle for urine so that the act of voiding is as independent as possible.
If he has more than one accident daily, go back to Step 3. Emphasize nonjudgmentally that the step back is temporary.	This procedure purposefully emphasizes a low-key approach. Bladder control can become ammunition for a battle between staff and patient if incontinence is viewed as staff failure or patient vengeance.
	Continence can determine whether a handicapped person goes home or to another institution following discharge from the rehabilitation hospital. A program that leads to continence is vital therapy.
	The patient may become 'nurse continent'—the nurse initiates toileting, anticipates for the patient. True continence is patient-initiated toileting which the patient 'times' so it does not interfere with other activities.
B. Recording 1. When therapy is instituted, write nursing order and enter on Kardex under problem and approaches.	
2. Evaluate effectiveness at patient-centered conferences and note in the progress notes.	

amounts in any one patient. One determines which are least impaired, and uses those to reinforce the patient's successful endeavors. The point is that we want this person to receive his input and to respond constructively.

MEMORY DEFICITS

To evaluate the information one receives, one must be able to scan the volume of memory data and select previous experiences that bear on the information now being received. Therapy for a memory deficit is aimed at helping the person recall past events and put them, and himself, in proper sequence. This is done by orienting him to person, place, and time.

For example, the day of the week is really an abstract concept. Tuesday is merely a word. But if Tuesday is the day one's mother visits, the word has more meaning. By the same token, times of day can be remembered best when they are presented in terms of events that occur at those times.

Attention to an activity can be personalized in the same way. The patient with a severe memory impairment is more likely to remember the time he sees Mary Ann, his physical therapist, than the time he has an appointment for physical therapy. The therapist's name, then, is used to designate the activity.

Another method of stimulating memory is to help the patient list his activities for the day. These notations can then be a basis for conversation with him. This eliminates the need to rely on his recall, which may reinforce error. As much as possible, the person's daily activities should be planned in an exact sequence each day. Predictable events are easier to remember. The patient's ability to predict also reduces his anxiety.

Loss of memory for recent events is common. Memory of distant past events may be virtually intact. Because the patient forgets, personnel must reintroduce themselves again and again. It is helpful if personnel on the unit wear tags giving the name by which they are called—If everyone calls Ms. Jones "Carol," then that should be the only name written on her tag.

Forgetting events is also a common problem, and must be accepted nonjudgmentally. For example, a patient may insist that he has not eaten shortly after meals have been served. He needs help to find his own method of reminder.

A primary goal in treating a patient who has difficulty remembering is to help him recognize and admit that very fact. He must be aware of some memory loss in order to see his need to rely on memory aids, such as lists and notes. Family teaching is essential with regard to the patient's memory loss and should, if possible, be undertaken before the symptom is observed. It particularly upsets relatives when the patient does not remember them or forgets that they visit him daily.

The patient's short memory may also interfere with aspects of his physical care. He will often pull out a nasogastric tube or remove a dressing because he cannot remember their purpose. Inconsistent memory must be dealt with at another level, too. It is necessary to validate the patient's word on occasion, and the more alert individual may interpret this validation as questioning his truthfulness. He needs to deal openly with his difficulty in remembering certain things, and gentle reminders that his memory is sometimes unreliable.

Once the patient's memory, reinforced by the staff's assistance, becomes dependable and he can be secure in the knowledge, for example, that his physical therapy appointment is at 10 o'clock each morning, his attention to other things can increase.

MAKING DECISIONS

As memory returns, decisions can be made on the basis of what is remembered. Adults who have had head injuries usually have impaired judgment, or difficulty in comparing the requirements of a task with their ability to meet these requirements. They often have difficulty relating their actions to their physical limitations. Here, again, intervention is necessary to ensure the patient's safety while helping him to become aware of his disabilities. Rely on observation of actual performance rather than assume that a deficit exists on the basis of the location of the injury.

Poor spatial perceptions can become a safety hazard which the staff must overcome by anticipating situations in which the patient may make poor decisions. If he is unable to evaluate his ability to transfer from bed to wheelchair by himself, the chair should not be at his bedside. If he cannot hold a water pitcher securely to get himself a drink, it should not be left within his reach. One must be alert to the potential problems in the patient's environment and not present challenges that are beyond him.

Because judgment is such a complex function, it is often the faculty that is permanently impaired even in the individual who has had relatively mild trauma. Staff members in a rehabilitation facility must be on guard constantly to provide for safety and good care. At the same time, they must allow the person maximum opportunities to exercise his judgment and make decisions that are within his capabilities.

Impaired judgment, which may appear as childlike simplicity or daredevil recklessness, and other symptoms of brain dysfunction are usually difficult for the lay person to deal with. Often, more support and teaching is necessary to help family and friends accept impaired cognition than paralysis of limbs. But these handicaps are part of severe head injuries and cannot be treated successfully if they are considered as separate entities.

Awareness of where the person is and sensitivity in finding ways to enable him to use his capabilities to compensate for his cognitive and physical limitations enhances rehabilitation efforts.

A Paraplegic Reflects....

RAY BURRIDGE

This young paralegic's reflections reveal why such patients may rebuff others' attempts to help them emotionally.

I opened my eyes and looked around. I was in a strange room, a strange bed, with strange things all around. A pint of blood and a bottle of clear liquid hung beside my bed with tubes that led into my arm. Other tubes seemed to come out of my throat and my chest.

Where was I? What happened? All I remembered was driving with three buddies from Canada to the States for a long weekend. It was Friday night and I was in the back seat of the car falling asleep.

A nurse in the room came over. I started to ask her what had happened—I couldn't talk! She told me I had been in a serious accident and had been thrown out of the car. I was in a hospital in Spokane, Washington. It was Wednesday. I couldn't talk because I had had a tracheostomy, but would be able to talk when the tube was removed. I had been unconscious for four days, had split my head open, had cuts to my face, eight broken ribs, a punctured and collapsed lung, and a broken collar bone. I had fractured my back and was paralyzed from the waist down. *What!*

I threw back the covers and tried to move. I couldn't! I closed my eyes and everything blanked out. I couldn't focus on anything. I cried, not from pain—I had none except in my shoulder—but from a lost, empty feeling.

MR. BURRIDGE *is an accountant with Alberta Wheat Pool, Calgary, Alberta, Canada. He writes, "I learned that to make it in society, I had to look through others' eyes. They aren't going to come knocking on your door."*

The nurse was still there when I opened my eyes. She had brought a pad and pencil so I could communicate. My first question, "Will I walk again?" she could not answer. She didn't know. We would have to wait and see the x-rays. "How long?" brought another evasive answer. The trach tube and chest tube would be removed in time.

"What about the other passengers in the car?" One fellow had a bruised shoulder, another a black eye and two cracked ribs. Both had remained in hospital overnight for observation and then had returned home. The driver of the car had been thrown out. He had received head injuries and would be in hospital for about 12 days. This information was no help. I could only think, *Why did I get so smashed up when they were hardly hurt at all? Why me?*

I was 400 miles from home and didn't know anyone. My parents had come down the night of the accident but I was unconscious and they returned home the next day. They were phoned again when I woke up and mom flew in that afternoon. At last I felt some security having someone I knew and could lean on for support. She told me how bad the accident had been. After I was admitted to the hospital and worked on for seven hours, a priest was called in to administer last rites. A chill went through my body. Why hadn't I just died when I was that close? What good was I? A cripple—not good for anything. I'd have to be taken care of all the time.

These thoughts recurred many times during the months that followed. I never considered suicide—I just wished I had died and that it was all over. I felt too weak to face the future.

Because I am unmarried and have lived on my own for over eight years, learning to be dependent was the first adjustment I had to accept. It was hard. I thought of all the things I could no longer do—swimming, horseback riding, hiking, dancing, traveling. Why wasn't I dead?

I was confused, I had no perspective on anything. Everyone had advice but none of it seemed to make sense and I did not want to hear their thoughts. Their ideas didn't coincide with mine and it seemed they were just trying to make conversation. I didn't appreciate people telling me what *they* thought I could still do. I wanted someone there for company—not to talk, just to be there.

Self-pity had not yet passed but I began facing facts. A nurse, my mother, and I discussed what I had to look forward to: a long period of bed rest, a longer stretch of physio-therapy to develop my upper body so I would be confident enough to do everything with my arms, including some things I used to use my legs for. Eventually I would leave the hospital and go out into society.

After 10 days in the American hospital, my trach and chest tubes were removed and I was flown to Foothills Hospital in Calgary. Once I was back in my home town I had many visitors, but soon I began to feel like a spectacle—a sideshow with everyone standing around and looking. Conversations got monotonous: "You are looking real good for what you have been through." "We are all pulling for you." "You'll make it. You've got what it takes." But these were just words. How could they know what it takes? It was fine for them. A half-hour visit and they could leave my room and return to their normal lives while I lay in bed trying to get my legs to move again. I began to resent visitors. I could predict what they were going to say. They had no idea of what a strain it was for me to be pleasant. I was torn inside when they mentioned something they had done and here I was, a hopeless cripple.

I went through two months of bed rest and then a back fusion operation and another four weeks of just lying in bed. Eventually I was allowed up in a wheelchair, and a week later I was transferred to a rehabilitation center for physiotherapy.

I felt so helpless, like a newborn baby with an adult mind. I had to learn to do everything I could do before, but in a different way. Simple things I once did with no effort or thought—getting out of bed, dressing, putting on a pair of shoes, making a cup of coffee—now became real chores.

After 17 weeks of hospitalization, I was getting very tired of hospital surroundings. When I received the news that I would be allowed to go out on a weekend pass, I was excited and scared. I looked forward to getting back to my apartment and things that were familiar. But the weekend was utter chaos! I had to be carried up the six front steps. I couldn't get through the bathroom door—my wheelchair was too wide. My bed was too low. Because of the furniture arrangement I couldn't get around easily. I felt disappointed and depressed.

When I returned to the hospital my therapist told me I was doing well and could probably leave the hospital soon. The news put me in a real panic. How could I leave?

Three weeks later I took another weekend pass. With adjustments made in my apartment—bricks under the legs of my bed, a narrower wheelchair so I could use the washroom, rearrangement of furniture—I was able to spend an enjoyable weekend away from hospital. My brother spent the weekend with me just in case I ran into difficulties. I still felt helpless and useless because I needed someone around all the time.

During successive weekends I tried to learn new ways of doing things. Then I met someone in the hospital who had been a paraplegic for two years. Meeting and talking to him was much better than trying to talk to a healthy person. Doctors, nurses, and therapists tried to put themselves in my place but it was beyond them. The emotional collapse and rebuilding necessary can't be imagined. Meeting someone who had the same limitations I had and hearing and seeing what he could do changed my attitude. If he could do it, so could I.

I began to look forward to leaving the hospital. With the assistance of a home service representative at the hospital I was able to rent a suitable house. I ordered a new car, a two-door sedan with a bench seat that would be adapted with hand controls. Finally, after nearly seven months in the hospital, I was discharged and moved into my new home with a friend.

I've had to cope with many problems since then—some people are over-solicitous, others ask rude and embarrassing questions. My former friends say they're too busy to spend time with me. I've come a long way, but I've learned that life as paraplegic is more than not being able to walk. It means restructuring your whole life—socially and emotionally, as well as physically.

Autonomic Hyperreflexia

DELYCIA FEUSTEL

A distended bladder or rectum can cause the spinal cord injured patient's blood pressure to rise to dangerous levels.

Autonomic hyperreflexia is one of the most serious emergencies that can develop during the rehabilitation of the person with spinal cord injury(1). Also called autonomic dysreflexia, this entity was first described by Head and Riddoch in 1917 as a "mass-reflex" that occurred below the level of a spinal cord lesion(2).

An excessive autonomic response to normal stimuli, autonomic hyperreflexia is characterized by paroxysmal hypertension, throbbing headache, blurred vision, sweating below the level of the lesion, bradycardia, nasal congestion, nausea, and pilomotor spasm(3,4). The onset of symptoms varies greatly, depending on the return of reflex function in the patient's spinal cord.

According to Kurnick, autonomic hyperreflexia occurs in persons with spinal cord lesions above most of the sympathetic nerve out-flow from the spine. Because the major splanchnic outflow comes from the fourth or sixth thoracic segment to the second lumbar segment of the spinal cord, autonomic dysfunction results from lesions above this level(5). However, Moeller states that hyperreflexia may be found in persons with lesions below the sixth thoracic segment, even at the eighth thoracic segment(6).

Autonomic hyperreflexia is triggered by visceral distention or contraction, particularly in the urinary bladder or rectum; stimulation of pain receptors; and stimulation of the skin(4). Thus, acute genitourinary

DELYCIA FEUSTEL, *R.N., M.S., is a clinical specialist in the nursing care of spinal cord injured persons, Texas Institute for Rehabilitation and Research, Houston.*

infections and distention of the intestine may trigger the reflex(7). Although symptoms are initiated by visceral or cutaneous stimuli or both anywhere below the level of cord injury, the genito-anal area is the most sensitive. The reflex can be initiated by distention of the renal pelvis, operative incisions below the level of the lesion, sharp touch, pressure on the glans penis causing the bulbocavernous reflex, or pressure on the testicle(3). Ejaculation in the man also can initiate the reflex as can strong uterine contractions in the pregnant woman. Symptoms generally appear when the patient's bladder tone and contractility return(8).

When sensory receptors below the level of the spinal cord lesion are stimulated, afferent impulses travel to the lower spinal cord and ascend in the lateral funiculi to the level of the cord lesion(4). The lesion blocks the afferent impulses from traveling up the spinothalamic tracts and posterior columns. Because the autonomic reflex, which is mediated through the lateral horn cells in the spinal cord, is intact, a reflex arteriolar spasm takes place in the skin and viscera. The increased sympathetic response causes the blood pressure to rise and profuse sweating below the level of the lesion(3,4).

The resulting hypertension is detected by the baroreceptors in the carotid sinus, aortic arch, and cerebral vessels. These receptors stimulate the ninth and tenth cranial nerves to carry afferent impulses to the vasomotor center of the medulla(3). Normally, this would set off a reaction causing efferent impulses of the tenth cranial nerve to go to the sinoatrial node of the heart to slow the cardiac rate. And other fibers would stimulate the splanchnic nerves to dilate the peripheral and visceral vasculature, thereby lowering the blood pressure.

However, in the person with a spinal cord lesion above the sympathetic outflow, these responses are somewhat altered. The efferent impulses along the tenth cranial nerve produce bradycardia, but the impulses to the sympathetic motor preganglionic neurons in the thoracic and lumbar segments cannot go beyond the spinal cord lesion. The result is that compensatory vasodilatation cannot occur below the lesion and severe hypertension persists even though vasodilatation occurs above the level of the lesion(4).

Patients who have middle and lower thoracic lesions are more likely to maintain homeostasis because the compensatory mechanism working in the upper part of the body is sufficient to control the symptoms below the lesion. However, in high thoracic and cervical lesions, the compensatory mechanism may be unable to prevent the sharp rise of blood pressure(9). If left untreated, the hypertension can cause loss of consciousness, epileptic seizures, cerebral hemorrhage, and death(5,7,9).

Autonomic hyperreflexia produces a variety of symptoms, either singly or in combination. For example, vasodilation still occurs above the lesion and results in hot, red skin, while vasoconstriction is the response below the lesion, resulting in pallor. The patient's pulse may become slow, irregular, and forceful and his blood pressure may climb precipitously, with a systolic reading as high as 240 to 300 mm. Hg(5,6). A person with an incomplete lesion, one that does not transsect the cord, might complain of discomfort in his abdomen, suprapubic region, or penis. He may experience chest pressure and difficulty breathing and complain about a headache which is located either in the occipital area or between his eyes(8). The person with a complete lesion usually would experience discomfort only above the level of the lesion.

Removing the triggering stimulus is the emergency treatment of acute hyperreflexia. In addition, the hospitalized patient needs to be taught the signs and symptoms of hyperreflexia so that he can notify the nurse when the symptoms first appear.

As soon as the signs and symptoms of hyperreflexia are noted, check the patient's blood pressure and then elevate the head of his bed 45 degrees to help lower his blood pressure. Monitor pressure and associated symptoms every five minutes as you proceed.

Check the patient's catheter to be sure it is not kinked or clogged, allowing urine to accumulate and distend the bladder. Next, irrigate the catheter; if no urine returns, remove it and insert a new catheter. Even the patient who does not have a catheter may have a distended bladder and need catherterization to reduce the pressure.

Other stimuli that can be removed or stopped promptly include any sharp object against his skin, a draft of cold air, or the movement of linen over his legs.

If the stimulus is a fecal impaction, do not attempt to remove it because this could cause more sympathetic stimulation and increase the patient's blood pressure. Before inserting a suppository to remove an impaction from any patient prone to develop autonomic hyperreflexia, the nurse should apply Nupercaine ointment (dibucaine HC1) to the anus and one inch into the rectum.

Pharmacological intervention may be necessary if the triggering stimulus cannot be removed. Pearman and England state that hyperreflexia can be stopped by blocking the sympathetic receptors or the alpha adrenergic receptors. For sudden acute hyperreflexia in an adult, they suggest diazoxide (Hyperstat I.V.) 300 mg. given by rapid intravenous injection. Failure to reduce the blood pressure is usually due to giving too small a dose or to administering it too slowly. The drug may be repeated at one-half to three-hour intervals with no more than four injections in 24 hours.

For chronic episodes of the vascular symptoms of hyperreflexia, a continuous alpha-adrenergic block, phenoxybenzamine (Dibenzyline) 10 to 20 mg., may be given every night or guanethidine sulfate (Ismelin) 10 mg. twice daily initially, with an average maintenance dose of 20 to 40 mg. per day(3). Since Ismelin is an adrenergic blocking agent, it does not affect the cholinergic receptors in the sweat glands. Also, Ismelin has a cumulative effect, so that it takes three to five days to become fully effective(10).

Sweating can be prevented with the cholinergic blocking medication propantheline bromide (Pro-Banthine) 30 to 45 mg. P.O. daily or one hour before manual evacuation of the rectum(4). However, Pro-Banthine also may affect the neurogenic bladder, causing urinary retention(3).

The first approaches to controlling this reflex were described in 1948 by Thompson who suggested a tetraethyl ammonium chloride nerve block, since analgesics and sedatives were ineffective, and then surgical sympathectomy(7). In 1956, Kurnick discouraged the use of such neurosurgical procedures as sacral neurotomy, sympathectomy, and subarachnoid alcohol injections because these approaches jeopardized the potential for bladder training, deprived the person of sexual potency, and were irreversible. Instead, he recommended using hexamethonium, a relatively long-acting ganglionic blocking agent which permitted bowel and bladder training(5).

The entire nursing staff must be aware of which patient has hyperreflexia, the usual triggering stimulus, and how to relieve the symptoms. If a patient has had one episode of hyperreflexia, he very likely will have more. His chart should be marked, much as is the allergic patient's, so that all staff are alerted to his problem.

The spinal cord injured person who is admitted to the rehabilitation center while in spinal shock does not need to know about hyperreflexia initially, since he may not have a spinal cord injury. However, the patient admitted with a spinal cord injury which is not in the shock phase is treated differently. During the initial nursing assessment, I determine how much the patient knows about hyperreflexia, whether or not he has had any of the symptoms, and, if so, what was done. Those who do not know about hyperreflexia are instructed.

I explain that the symptoms are mild initially and that the blood pressure elevations are slight. However, I do explain that blood pressure levels increase with each episode so that it is important to detect this reaction early. I reassure them that there is medication to control the blood pressure, that the reaction may be a one-time occurrence, and that the patient may never have hyperreflexia.

All patients are checked periodically until it is clear that they understand the necessary information. When a patient has a hyperreflexic episode, the nurse should discuss the symptoms with the patient and family so they can be prepared for any future episodes. Before discharge, the patient is instructed not only about symptoms but also about possible sources of stimuli and what to do to interrupt them. Each spinal cord injured person who has had or who is susceptible to hyperreflexia receives a home instruction booklet.

The experience of an 18-year-old quadriplegic man who had two episodes of hyperreflexia illustrated the care described. His injury was at the level of the fifth and sixth cervical spines. Two and a half months after he had a cervical fusion, he was given bethanechol (Urecholine) 2.5 mg. subcutaneously to increase bladder contractility. He immediately developed red patches on his chest, upper arms, and face. His blood pressure rose from a normal 100/60 to 140/100. He was given Ismelin 10 mg. P.O. and catheterized. One hour later his blood pressure was 130/80 and his skin clear.

One month after this episode with Urecholine, he had a similar experience when he received a bisacodyl (Dulcolax) suppository. The suppository was given at 8 P.M. and a half hour later, his skin again became red and blotchy, he perspired, and complained of a throbbing headache. His blood pressure was 145/105. He was given Ismelin 10 mg. P.O. and his fecal impaction was removed.

His blood pressure peaked at 172/108 at 2 A.M. the next morning, but returned to 120/80 by 8 A.M. He was placed on a maintenance dose of Ismelin 5 mg. orally three times a day and Nupercaine ointment to rectum before inserting any suppository. After being on Ismelin four days, his only hyperreflexic symptom was perspiration at the time of his bowel movement.

The patient and those caring for him must understand that hyperreflexia can occur in any patient whose spinal cord injury occurs above the sympathetic nerve outflow. And it is the nurse's quick action to remove the triggering stimulus that can save this patient.

REFERENCES
1. SELL, G. H., AND OTHERS. Autonomic hyperreflexia and catecholamine metabolites in spinal cord injury. *Arch.Phys.Med.Rehabil.* 53:415-417, 424, Sept. 1972.
2. HEAD, H., AND RUDDOCH, J. Automatic bladder, excessive sweat-

ing and some other reflex conditions in gross injuries. *Brain* 40:188-263, 1917.
3. SHEA, J. D., AND OTHERS. Autonomic hyperreflexia in spinal cord injury. *South.Med.J.* 66:869-872, Aug. 1973.
4. PEARMAN, J. W., AND ENGLISH, E. J. *Urological Management of the Patient Following Spinal Cord Injury.* Springfield, Ill., Charles C Thomas, Publisher, 1973.
5. KURNICK, N. B. Autonomic hyperreflexia and its control in patients with spinal cord lesions. *Ann.Intern.Med.* 44:678-686. April. 1956.
6. MOELLER, B. A., AND SCHEINBERG, D. Autonomic dsyreflexia in injuries below the sixth thoracic segment. *JAMA*. 224:1295, May 28, 1973.
7. THOMPSON, C. E., AND WITHAM, A.C. Paroxysmal hypertension in the spinal cord injury. *N.Engl.J.Med.* 239:291-294, Aug. 19, 1948.
8. GUTTMANN, N. LUDWIG. Spinal Cord Injuries; Comprehensive Management and Research. Oxford. Blackwell Scientific Publications, 1973.
9. GUTTMAN, LUDWIG, AND WHITTERIDGE, D. Effects of bladder distention on autonomic mechanisms after spinal cord injuries. *Brain* 70:364-404, 1947.
10. GOODMAN, L. S., AND GILMAN, ALFRED. *The Pharmacological Basis of Therapeutics.* 4th ed. New York, Macmillan Company, 1970, pp. 572-573.

Sexual Function in Traumatic Paraplegia and Quadriplegia

A. ESTIN COMARR • BERNICE B. GUNDERSON

Determining the extent of the patient's spinal lesion is the all-important first step in helping both patient and partner gradually achieve a satisfactory sexual adjustment.

Recently there has been a marked upswing of interest in the sexual potential of spinal-cord-injured patients. Study groups have been formed, lectures and seminars presented, and counseling and research initiated to help the person with paraplegia or quadriplegia and his partner adjust to their sexual roles.

The essential first steps are a careful neurological examination of the patient and an interview with him and his sexual partner to ascertain exactly what sexual potential the injured person has. Once this has been clearly documented, all those who work with the patient have a better chance of coping realistically.

LEVEL AND EXTENT OF INJURY

The neurophysiological aspects of sexual function have been reviewed by Bors and Comarr[1]. Several statistical studies have been published concerning sex among relatively large groups of patients with traumatic cord and/or cauda equina lesions[1,2,5,6,8-11]. Three original studies

---

DR. COMARR *received his M.D. degree from Chicago Medical School, Chicago, Ill. He is currently an attending urologist at Rancho Los Amigos Hospital, Downey, California.* MS. GUNDERSON *graduated from White Memorial Hospital School of Nursing, Los Angeles, Calif., and received her B.S. degree from Loma Linda University, Loma Linda, Calif. She is currently supervising nurse of the genitourinary service at Rancho Los Amigos Hospital.*

by one of the authors are based on neurological findings and segmental levels of injury(1,2,5,6); other large studies (8-11) are based on the vertebral levels of injury. Just as we have classified the traumatic cord bladder based on whether reflex activity is or is not present from the second through fourth sacral segments of the spinal cord, so we have classified sexual function among these patients. The diagnosis is made by digital rectal examination.

The presence of tone in the external (striated) rectal sphincter, a positive bulbocavernosus reflex, or both indicate that the patient has an upper motor neuron lesion and is capable of reflex sexual function. The absence of external rectal-sphincter tone, an absent bulbocavernosus reflex, or both indicate that the patient has lower motor neuron involvement and is capable of areflexic sexual function. To ascertain whether the cord lesion is complete or incomplete—that is, whether it does or does not transect the spinal cord—at the S2 though S4 segments, the penile skin, scrotal skin, and saddle area are tested bilaterally with a pin prick to determine whether the spinothalamic (sensory) and posterior (motor) column pathways are intact.

The followng findings are characteristic of the four types of lesions described above:

1. *complete upper motor neuron lesion:* no sensation or volitional control of the external rectal spincter in the presence of external rectal sphincter tone, a positive bulbocavernosus reflex, or both.

2. *incomplete upper motor neuron lesion:* only light touch sensation or partial loss of pin prick sensation, and the loss of volitional control of the external rectal sphincter in the presence of external rectal sphincter tone, a positive bulbocavernosus reflex, or both.

3. *complete lower motor neuron lesion:* no sensation, volitional control, or tone of the external rectal sphincter, and no bulbocavernosus reflex.

4. *incomplete lower motor neuron lesion:* partial sensation but no volitional control of the external rectal sphincter, no external rectal sphincter tone, and no bulbocavernosus reflex.

SEXUAL CAPABILITY

Based on this neurological classification, statistical studies (1,2,5,6) and reviews (3,4) can be summarized thus:

The majority of men with *upper motor neuron lesions* have reflexogenic erections either spontaneously at any time or in response to external stimulation applied to the penis, such as manual massage, pulling the catheter, pulling the external urinary receptacle, fellatio, and so forth. A reflexogenic erection is produced by reflex activity, spontaneously and by external stimulation.

Those patients who can attain reflexogenic erections only spontaneously are unfortunate in that these erections can occur at any time during the day or night, but may not be attainable when actually wanted, and may be of such short duration that coitus is impossible.

Some patients who attain reflexogenic erections by external stimulation may not be able to consummate coitus because the erection may be fleeting. Some patients with upper motor neuron lesions never have an erection.

About 70 percent of men with complete lesions can consummate coitus, whereas the percentage is higher—80 percent or more—for those with incomplete lesions. Successful coitus implies not only intromission but that the woman reaches an orgasm.

The vast majority of men with *complete upper motor neuron lesions* cannot ejaculate or have an orgasm, and consequently cannot sire children. The hyperactivity of the sacral segments seems to inhibit ejaculation among patients with complete lesions. However, there are some exceptions in a very few patients whose injury is at the visceral outflow of the splanchnic nerves and below the tenth thoracic level. Possibly these patients' lesions which appear clinically complete are not anatomically complete. Perhaps these few exceptional men have not told the truth during interviews, or perhaps the autonomic nervous system is playing a role in these discrepancies.

Whether the patient with an *incomplete* upper motor neuron lesion will ejaculate and sire children depends on the extent of the lesion. The smaller the neurological deficit, the greater the chance for psychogenic erections and ejaculations.

Among men with *complete lower motor neuron lesions*, about 75 percent are unable to have erections of any kind, and, therefore, unable to have coitus, ejaculation, orgasm, or to sire children. About 25 percent can have psychogenic erections, which are produced by mental, or mental and physical, stimuli. These patients have segmental lesions below T-12. Of the patients with psychogenic erections, a smaller number will be able to consummate coitus because of non-firm or too brief erections, and fewer men still can ejaculate.

Among patients with *incomplete lower motor neuron lesions,* as many as 83 percent may have psychogenic erections, with a 90 percent successful rate of coitus. Fifty percent to 70 percent of this group may be able to ejaculate. Ten percent of those who can ejaculate may sire children. That this 10 percent has the highest potential for procreation becomes

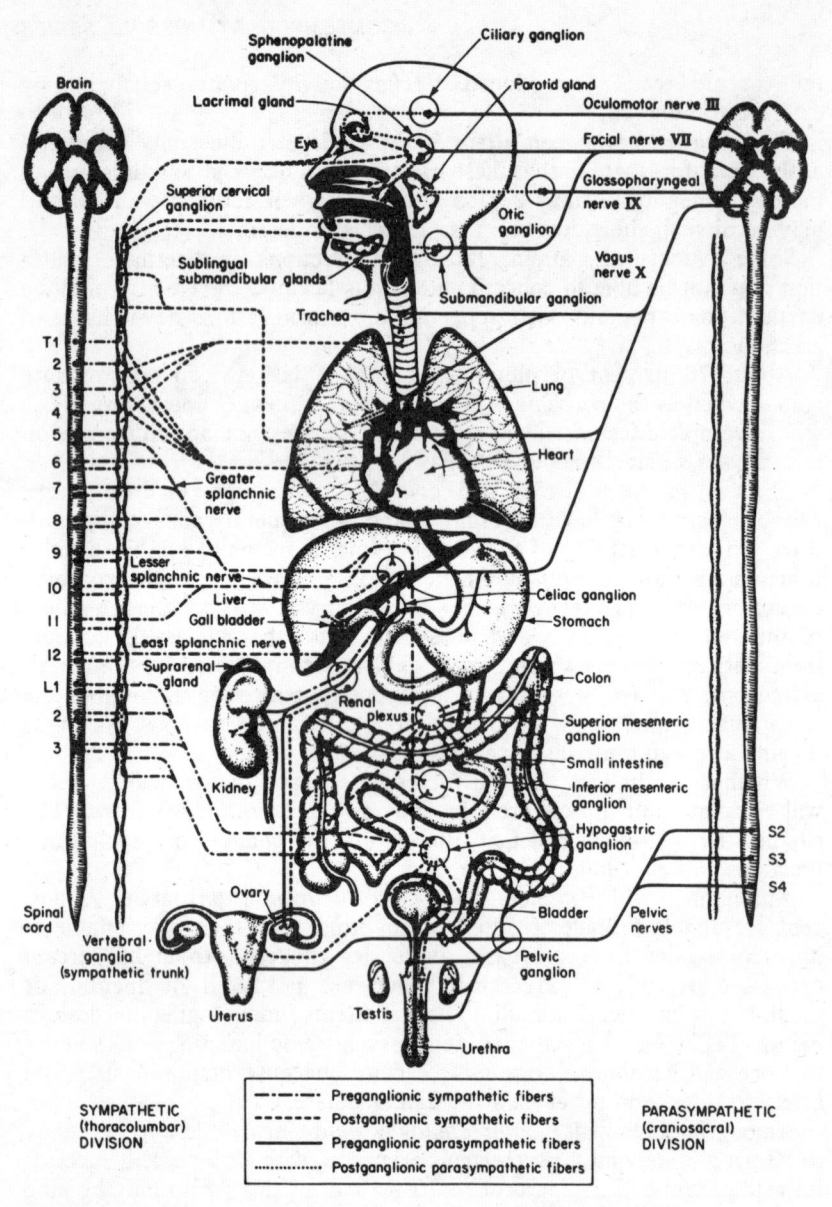

The degree of motor and sensory loss depends on the extent and location of the spinal cord injury.

obvious when one notes that in a series of 529 patients studied, irrespective of level, only three percent sired children(1).

The woman who has paraplegia or tetraplegia and is of childbearing age usually regains menses(5,6). Nearly 50 percent do not miss a single period. The ability to have an orgasm is usually lost, but the majority of female patients do continue sexual activity. Irrespective of injury level—cervical, thoracic, lumbar, or sacral—women have the potential to become pregnant. If their pelvic measurements are adequate, most women can have vaginal deliveries. Urinary tract complications seem to occur more frequently among paralyzed primiparas, than among nonparalyzed women.

Heretofore the literature has presented case histories of patients only. To substantiate the accuracy of each patient's statements, we interviewed the partner. Nine case histories are presented here. A careful neurological examination was done for each patient, and the patient and partner were interviewed separately so that both could speak freely.

CASE HISTORIES

Mr. and Ms. C. are both 39 years of age. They have three school-age children who are living at home. Mr. C. was injured in a fall from a scaffold, and sustained a complete paraplegia at the T-8 level. Although one would expect a spastic, or upper motor neuron, paralysis from injury at this level, Mr. C. has a flaccid, or lower motor neuron, paralysis due to secondary cord degeneration. He voids by straining and is able to empty his bladder completely. Bowel management is by manual evacuation.

Mr. C. was well-developed muscularly and very strong before injury. His rehabilitation progressed so rapidly that he became independent in a relatively short time. However, as is often true, his physical rehabilitation was complete before his psychological adjustment was achieved. Rather than returning home, he went to a second rehabilitation hospital. After several months there, he finally could accept going home. At the time of our interview, one and one-half years after injury, Mr. C. had not returned to work, although he was well qualified as a typist and could work conveniently from his wheelchair.

The C.'s sexual adjustment has been very difficult. Mr. C. cannot achieve an erection either psychogenically or reflexly, an intolerable blow to one who prided himself on his sexual ability before injury. Shortly after discharge, he and his wife attempted intercourse on two occasions. Because of his strong arms, he could assume the dominant position and place the flaccid penis in his wife's vagina manually. Ms. C. accepted this and found the attempts satisfying. However, when she subsequently made sexual overtures, Mr. C. rebuffed her, saying that the experience was unrewarding for him and not worth the effort. This was so damaging to her ego that she decided never to approach him again and when he later tried to make amends and said he would try for "her sake," she rejected him. During the interview, Ms. C. talked about the problem and recognized the extent of her frustration. She had begun experiencing headaches and other physical symptoms. She had tried tranquilizers, but was afraid of becoming "hooked." She admitted that sexual experience outside the home was a possibility, but because of her strong religious background, she thought that guilt feelings would prevent any fulfillment. On one occasion, she went out to dinner with a male companion, but was unable to bring herself to go any further.

We were impressed that this couple was in real need of counseling and spent considerable time trying to help him adjust. We believe that a meaningful relationship is possible if a couple can be helped past a poor beginning. We suggested to Mr. C. that he "court" his wife again and that they gradually engage in touching and fondling without attempting genital contact. If they fail, it seems likely that the marriage will not endure.

Mr. and Ms. D. each sustained a spinal cord injury in the same auto accident 10 years ago. Mr. D., now 48 years old, is a paraplegic at the T-10 level and Ms. D., age 44, is a quadriplegic at the C-5 level. Mr. D's original injury, at the L-1 level, was the lower motor neuron flaccid type. Because he was severely incapacitated by pain, a cordotomy was performed. This raised the sensory (spinothalamic) level of paraplegia and alleviated some of his pain.

He has had a suprapubic catheter for 10 years. At no time since injury has he achieved any erection. Ms. D. has no feeling below the shoulders, including the nipple area, and cannot feel any response to sexual stimulation. She has had a urethral catheter since injury. Mr. and Ms. D's sexual life ended with the accident that paralyzed them. Mr. D. has noticed that her nipples become erect when stimulated, but she does not perceive any response. Even kissing, which previously stimulated her, no longer does so. Mr. and Ms. D. do not sleep together as she needs a hospital bed with a Balkan frame and loops for transferring to and from her wheelchair.

This couple has achieved a remarkable adjustment, but it did not come easily. Mr. D. is a musician and, after his cordotomy, he returned to full-time employment as a junior high school music director, even leading the school's marching band from his wheelchair. Shortly after Mr. D. returned to work, they decided to get along without a live-in attendant and Mr. D. assumed responsibility for undressing Ms. D. and putting her to bed at night. A day time attendant cares for her while Mr. D. is at work. Their two children remained at home and are now grown and successful. The parents participated in their care and activities as much as possible. The D.'s continue to be affectionate and responsive to each other and seem to have achieved the best possible relationship under the most trying conditions.

Ms. I. is a 28-year-old paraplegic with a segmentally complete lesion at the T-5 level on the right and T-6 level on the left. She was injured 20 years ago when she was pushed by a playmate from an overpass onto a freeway. She has worn a urethral catheter during this entire period. Her menstrual periods have always been regular.

In 1967, Ms. I. married a serviceman and they now have three children. Ms. I. stated at the interview that she found sexual relations very satisfying. The most pleasurable sensations come from breast stimulation, but she also enjoys clitoral and vaginal stimulation, either manual or penile. She was quite concerned about birth control methods because she was then pregnant with her third child. She had rejected the "pill," tried an intrauterine device which was unsatisfactory due to excessive menstrual flow and cramping, and Mr. I. had tried "withdrawal," which was also unsatisfactory. Subsequently, Mr. I. has had a vasectomy. A neurologically normal man, Mr. I. stated that his wife was very responsive to sexual overtures. During coitus her limbs become spastic and she develops cutis anserina, or goose flesh, over the lower abdomen and legs. These pleasurable responses may be interpreted as a "sexual equivalent" which seem normal to the patient because she had had no sexual experiences prior to incurring her injury.

Mr. I. stated that he enjoys sexual relations with his wife as much as he previously did with neurologically normal partners. At first, he found it necessary to remove his wife's catheter before coitus due to her narrow vagina, but since the delivery of their first child this has not been necessary. About 75 percent of the time Mr. I. assumes the usual dominant position during intercourse, but the other 25 percent of the time he assists her into the dominant position, and both positions seem equally pleasurable.

It appears that a very happy relationship is possible for a paraplegic woman, especially one without prior sexual experiences. The I.'s three children were all delivered vaginally. Ms. I.'s only complication was a kidney infection during her first pregnancy.

Mr. K. is a 32-year-old quadriplegic who was injured in a diving accident at the age of 15. He has no motor function below the C-7 level, but he has pin prick sensation to the T-5 dermatome on the left and T-4 on the right. Light touch is intact throughout his entire body, including penile and scrotal skin and saddle areas. He has no volitional control of the external rectal sphincter.

Mr. K. finished high school and college after his injury and subsequently was hired by a government agency as a tax consultant. He has had regular promotions, is now entirely self-supporting, and has even had a home constructed that is suited to his wheelchair existence.

At 28, Mr. K. married a co-worker. Neither he nor his wife had had previous sexual experiences. This fact probably made adaptation to the wife's assumption of the dominant position easier for them. Ms. K., rather slight of build, does not have the strength to pull her husband into the dominant position so they have never tried this.

Mr. K. wore an external appliance in the early years after his injury, but later developed a ureteral stricture and hydronephrosis which necessited using an indwelling Foley catheter. In addition, he is quite subject to autonomic dysreflexia and, therefore, hesitant to remove his catheter unnecessarily. Autonomic dysreflexia is an abnormal hypertensive response to stimuli, usually from the bladder or rectum, in patients who have spinal cord lesions above the T-6 level.

All Mr. K.'s efforts at coitus have been with the catheter in place and connected to the drainage container. The catheter folds back against the penis and does not interfere with sexual activity now, although it caused Ms. K. some discomfort at first. Mr. K. is able to achieve reflex erections with manual stimulation, usually by his wife. When first married, they attempted coitus once or twice daily and he could ejaculate only with additional manual stimulation. Now, however, the frequency of coitus has decreased to once weekly and he ejaculates spontaneously during intercourse about 75 percent of the time. Mr. and Ms. K. have noticed that his erections last longer when his legs are spastic and after instillation of Pontocaine solution into the bladder. Pontocaine is used to decrease symptoms of autonomic dysreflexia at catheter change.

It is quite unlikely that Ms. K. has ever achieved a climax. She enjoys her husband's pleasure, but how long this will satisfy her needs is questionable. Mr. K. has had high hopes of fathering a child. This is not entirely unrealistic as he is able to ejaculate. However, his best sperm count has been only 10,000,000 per cc., 30 percent being of normal morphology and 10 percent of normal motility.* The K.'s are now considering artificial insemination by donor sperm mixed with Mr. K's. In

---

*Normal sperm count: 60-150 million; 80% or more motile, and 80-90% normal morphology. *Cecil Loeb Textbook of Medicine.* 11th edition, edited by Paul B. Beeson and Walsh McDermott. Philadelphia, W. B. Saunders Co., 1963, p. 1835.

the meantime, they have adopted an infant son who has brought them much happiness.

Ms. P. is a 37-year-old quadriplegic woman who was injured in an auto accident in 1962. She was a speech therapist and had been married for only three months at the time of the accident. She has a complete lesion at the C-4 level. She has had an indwelling catheter since her injury.

According to Mr. P., his wife was rather shy and naive when he married her and she did not like manual genital stimulation. She responded to kissing and fondling of her breasts, however. After the injury she had no feeling in either her breasts or genitals and so they discarded all sexual foreplay. Mr. P. misses her response and realizes that she gets no satisfaction from coitus. Ms. P. does want to please her husband, however, and lets him know when she is ready for sexual relations by sticking out her tongue slightly when he approaches her. Mr. P. completes coitus much more rapidly than before Ms. P.'s injury and with considerably less frequency, ranging from once a week to once a month, depending on how she feels.

Three years after her injury this couple planned a pregnancy, and in 1966 she delivered a boy who was several weeks premature but otherwise healthy. She was delivered vaginally, with spinal anesthesia for control of autonomic dysreflexia. Five years later they planned another pregnancy, and in 1972 a girl was born, two months prematurely. This was also a normal vaginal delivery. The P.'s use the "pill" for birth control.

Coitus has always been performed with the catheter in place. Although the P.'s life is far from normal, they have adjusted well to a very difficult situation and, with the help of Ms. P.'s mother, they are able to enjoy their children.

E. V. has an incomplete cord injury at the C 5-6 level from a driving accident in 1963. He has weak volitional contraction and relaxation of the external sphincter by rectal examination, some movement in his right leg, feels light touch in the penis and scrotal skin, and may be somewhat hypalgesic.

E. V. was engaged at the time of injury and one year later he and his girlfriend were married. During his rehabilitation, his girlfriend learned how to care for him completely, including his bowel care and application of his external urinary device. Ms. V. says that her husband's accident in no way changed her feelings about him and that she never considered not going ahead with their marriage.

Mr. V. has erections, probably of reflexogenic origin, although Ms. V. thinks some may be psychogenic. About half the erections are spontaneous and half require manual stimulation, sometimes for as much as 30 minutes. Although E. V. does not have good bladder control, he knows when he is going to void reflexly and is able to withdraw so that he does not void into the vagina during intercourse. Ms. V. usually assumes the dominant position but, because she is quite strong, sometimes pulls him over into the dominant position.

Ms. V. feels that she achieves a climax at least part of the time, but Mr. V. is afraid she may not be getting full satisfaction. On one occasion about a year after injury, Mr. V. had an orgasm and ejaculated, but this has not occured since. The V.'s have sexual relations only about three times a month, but they seem to agree that their marriage holds many compensations and enjoyments other than sex.

Mr. and Ms. V. discussed his inability to father children and considered donor insemination. However, Mr. V. decided against this and Ms. V. has been able to accept this decision. Ms. V. has a full-time job as a secretary and Mr. V. baby sits for a neighbor at home. Neither of them seems to be upset by this apparent reversal of roles. The V.'s appear to have a very stable and happy marriage.

Mr. N. sustained an incomplete cervical injury of the Brown-Sequard type in March 1971. He regained function rapidly and by August 1971 was walking without braces. Pin prick sensation was intact in the sacral segments, but he did not have voluntary control of the rectal sphincter. He had precipitous micturition, could not voluntarily stop his stream when voiding, and had difficulty in distinguishing between flatus and bowel movements.

Although he could attain a psychogenic erection at will he was unable to ejaculate or have an orgasm. Ms. N. stated that she was satisfied each time and that her husband could now maintain an erection longer than he could before the injury.

Mr. N. was seen again in January 1972 and still was unable to ejaculate. He was advised to try manual and/or vibrator stimulation. This was not successful. He returned on March 31, 1972, one year after injury, and happily reported that two weeks before the visit he had begun to ejaculate normally. Neurological examination revealed that he had regained voluntary control of the external sphincters and had made an almost total recovery.

Mr. N.'s case demonstrates the advantages of conservative management and patience with the person who has an incomplete spinal lesion.

V. R. is a 25-year-old paraplegic who has a complete injury at the T-4 level. He is incontinent but has a balanced bladder, that is, the ratio of voided urine to residual urine is 4:1 or 3:1. He wears an external appliance. He had no sexual experiences prior to his injury at age 18 but he did have wet dreams. He can attain a reflex erection by manual manipulation and can complete intromission, but he cannot maintain the erection long enough to satisfy his partner. However, with continued manual stimulation he can ejaculate and have an orgasm, and he can bring his partner to climax by digital stimulation. Mr. R. is one of a small group of patients who, by all accepted neurological tests, have complete cord injuries but can still ejaculate.

Mr. L. was injured while driving in 1961, when he was 22. He has an incomplete cervical injury. Sensation to pin prick is intact in the penis, scrotal skin, and left side of the saddle area; absent in the right saddle area. He has no volitional control of the external sphincters and no leg movement, has never achieved a balanced bladder, and has worn a Foley catheter since injury.

Six years after his accident. Mr. L. married a young woman with no previous sexual experience. He, too, had had no sexual relations due to his strict religious upbringing. Mr. L. achieves reflex erections but these are not of long enough duration to make intercourse possible and they are painful. Manual or vibrator stimulation has not been helpful.

When the L.'s were first married Mr. L. was very interested in sex, and he and his wife developed a quite satisfactory relationship by practicing cunnilingus on a daily basis. Ms. L. stated that she achieved considerable satisfaction. Manual stimulation of the clitoris and vaginal areas was not as pleasurable to her.

As time went on, Mr. L. became less interested in sex and less willing to make efforts to satisfy his wife. Their sexual contact decreased to only once every two months. Mr. L. became active in school, church, and work activities and declared he was "too busy" to worry about sex which gave him no pleasure. Ms. L. believes that her husband is not interested in how she feels and she is very depressed about the situation. She would like to have a child but Mr. L is not willing to adopt and is lukewarm about artificial insemination. She can look into it if she wants to, he says, but he "doesn't have time."

It seems unlikely that this marriage can endure under the circumstances. Probably the couple's strong religious background has preserved it thus far. Efforts to counsel Mr. L. have not been fruitful. He looks on the marriage as advantageous to him because his wife cares for him. However, he is unwilling to change so as to meet her needs.

The diagnosis of sexual potential is based essentially on a somatic neurologic examination. Even though the exact status of the autonomic nervous system is unknown, this classification has proved to be practical for bedside or office examination and does not require expensive, time-consuming testing.

The majority of catheter-dependent patients remove their catheters for coitus and reintroduce them afterward. For convenience, however, many patients have intercourse without removing the catheter; it simply folds over the penis during intromission. Many patients perform coitus with their condoms, or external urine-collecting devices in place. Those who remove the indwelling catheter or condom should endeavor to empty the bladder before intercourse to prevent involuntary voiding into the vagina, which is esthetically offensive to some women. To date there has been no published evidence that urine in the vaginal tract has created pathology, perhaps because the woman is usually in the dominant position.

Fellatio and cunnilingus are practiced by many patients, and these oral techniques are being stressed by some groups. However, we believe that counselors should know what potential the patient has for genital sex and the attitudes and religious beliefs of the patient and his partner before discussing fellatio and cunnilingus.

The use of a vibrator has been helpful in producing ejaculation, essentially among persons with incomplete lesions, for whom coitus itself may not always be enough stimulus. A vibrator also may make an erection firm enough to achieve intromission.

In our experience, medication such as injectable testosterone is only rarely of value. Interestingly, time and patience have brought spontaneous returns of sexual function that could have been wrongly attributed to medication. We have seen people with cauda equina lesions who have had spontaneous returns after years of waiting. Metandren linguets (methyltestosterone) are not recommended because of potential damage to the liver.

Men who are unable to attain erections are informed regarding "stuffing technique" and manual clitoral stimulation as methods of satisfying their sexual partners. Perhaps there should be greater use of various prostheses among this group. The discussion must be *very tactfully* handled and undertaken only after the counselors have gained insight into the personalities of the individuals being counseled.

The inability to sire children troubles the majority of spinal-cord-injured patients and their wives. Spermatozoa for the artificial insemination of their wives have been retrieved from some men who cannot ejaculate, but live births have been rare(7). Further research in this field will probably be rewarding. At this time, adoption or donor insemination seem the more practical methods of achieving parenthood.

REFERENCES

1. BORS, E., AND COMARR, A. E. Neurological disturbances of sexual function with special reference to 529 patients with spinal cord injury. *Urol. Survey* 10:191-222, Dec. 1960.
2. COMARR, A. E. Sexual function among patients with spinal cord injury. *Urol. Int.* 25:134-168, 1970.
3. ───── Sexual concepts in traumatic cord and cauda equina lesions. *J.Urol.* 106:375-378, Sept. 1971.
4. ───── *Sex among patients with Spinal Cord and/or Cauda Equina Injuries.* (To be published)
5. ───── Observations on menstruation and pregnancy among female spinal cord injury patients. *Paraplegia* 3:263-272. Feb. 1966.
6. ───── Interesting observations among females with spinal cord injury. *Med.Serv.J. Canada* 22:651-661, July-Aug. 1966.
7. GUTTMAN, N. L., AND OTHERS. Prostigmin assessment test of fertility in spinal man. *Paraplegia* 9:39-51, May 1971.
8. TABOT, H. S. Report on sexual function in paraplegia. *J.Urol.* 61:265-270. Feb. 1949.
9. ───── Sexual function in paraplegia. *J. Urol.* 73:91-100, Jan. 1955.
10. TSUJI, L., AND OTHERS. The sexual function in patients with spinal cord injury. *Urol. Int.* 12:270-280, 1961.
11. ZEITLIN, A. B., AND OTHERS. Sexology of the paraplegic male. *Fertil. Steril.* 8:337-344, July-Aug. 1957.

Sexuality and the Severely Disabled Person

JIM SMITH • BONNIE BULLOUGH

The sex act itself is not the chief difficulty—the real problem is finding a suitable partner, say these authors.

Sex problems of the disabled person are just starting to receive attention in nursing literature. Perhaps nurses have thought that sexual problems were medical rather than nursing concerns. We believe that this is not so, and offer some specific suggestions for nurses who are interested in either primary or secondary sex counseling for disabled people.

Our information is based on personal experience and on interviews and observations of persons with cerebral palsy, muscular dystrophy, post-poliomyelitis neurological damage, and traumatic injuries. From these sources, as well as the literature, it seems safe to conclude that a major cause of frustration and anxiety among the severely disabled is fear of sexual inadequacy[1,2,3].

This fear is also a significant factor in the depression, or other symptoms, of a newly injured person, and even remains a nagging concern among some people who have been disabled from birth.

Feelings of sexual inadequacy contribute to the alienation of the disabled from the mainstream of society and increase their tendency to see themselves as members of a deviant subculture. Unfortunately, members

---

JIM SMITH, B.A., has been quadriplegic since a swimming pool accident in 1967. He has lectured on sexuality and the severely disabled, and has developed a sexuality program for disabled students at the University of California, Riverside. BONNIE BULLOUGH, R.N., PH.D., a well-known editor and author, is a professor of nursing at California State University, Long Beach, and associate professor in residence at the California College of Medicine, Univ. of California, Irvine.

of the health care team have been largely unaware of these concerns, as the following incident suggests:

One day we convened a panel of wheelchair men for some of our residents. These men were in their twenties, and I was amazed to learn that if they had their choice between getting back their walking or their normal sexual function, they'd choose sex—it was that important to them. In the hospital we put all our effort toward the walking—we were doing nothing about this other problem.(4)

Since hospitals and rehabilitation centers are the primary institutions of resocialization for newly disabled people, their staffs have a responsibility to help patients lead a life as close to normal as possible. Unfortunately, even the most progressive staff members in these institutions have tended to shrink from this responsibility when it came to sex, or have left all sex counseling to physicians, ignoring the potential contributions of other workers.

THE PARADOX

This situation is paradoxical, considering that centers for the rehabilitation of patients with spinal cord injuries have some of the best team workers in patient care. The physical and occupational therapists, nurses, social workers, and others are all crucial in helping patients to become self-sufficient. Yet sex counseling has remained, by default, almost exclusively in the purview of physicians who, for various reasons, may not always be the best qualified to carry out this function. They bring a physiological bias to a problem that is really as much social as physiological. For example, a leading rehabilitation authority states:

I prefer only superficial counseling of the patient during the early months after injury and request that the patient discuss his sexual situation after he has been home and made attempts at coitus. Knowing what the patient can or cannot do aids the physician in making appropriate helpful suggestions.(5)

From a purely physiological standpoint, this is reasonable advice. Immediately following a spinal injury, there is a period of decreased reflex activity below the level of the injury and the muscles are flaccid. This period is often termed "spinal shock." A Babinski and other pathological reflexes may appear within a day or so, but complete recovery of normal reflex activity below the injury may take as long as six weeks.

For this reason, an accurate evaluation of the extent of the injury may not be possible until that time(6). Moreover, even when the extent of the injury is known, it is still impossible to be certain about sexual function, so the prudent diagnostician may well want to avoid making prognostic statements.

Psychologically, however, superficial counseling, such as telling a patient to report back when he has tried coitus, has some negative consequences. The person is likely to get the impression that sex is a taboo subject with health professionals, so he will be unlikely to share concerns with them. And such advice implies that only those persons who have loving mates waiting at home will have any sexual interests and that disabled persons who do not already have partners will want to remain celibate for the rest of their lives. The fact is that large numbers of the newly disabled are unmarried and have no lovers.

Many of the disabled people we interviewed told us that once they were able to attempt sexual intercourse, they could experiment with positions or techniques until they found a way to achieve and give some measure of satisfaction. Given the opportunity, technical problems were not prohibitive. The real difficulty for most of them was to find a mate who was willing to work through the problems with them. The issue of sexual incompatibility is of secondary importance to the disabled person who does not have a partner. Most of the counseling that is done is superficial because it fails to come to grips with this crucial issue. It misses its mark by taking a purely physiological approach rather than addressing the human social problems which are involved.

THE PRIMARY SEX COUNSELOR

More often than not, disabled persons are given no sex counseling. In a follow-up study of 47 patients with various types of myelopathy who had been seen in a large urban rehabilitation center, 77 percent of the men and 90 percent of the women reported that they had received no sex counseling from any health professional(7).

We propose two types of help. First, a primary sex counselor is needed who will take responsibility for seeing that the patient gets the assistance and support he or she needs. Second, the person should be given informal secondary support by other members of the health team, particularly if the primary counselor is of the opposite sex.

The primary counselor could be a physician, but might just as well be a sex therapist, clinical nurse specialist, psychologist, marriage counselor, or minister. Whoever takes on this responsibility should be suited by training and temperament. His or her preparation should include education about human interaction and the group process as well as the physiological and sociological aspects of sexuality.

CLIMATE OF COUNSELING SESSIONS

Under certain circumstances, it may be advantageous to employ a counselor who is himself disabled, although it is certainly possible for an empathetic, able-bodied person to do a creditable job. All counselors need to work through their personal sex problems, moral convictions, and values so that these are not imposed on clients. Sex therapists who work with disabled persons may also need to learn to accept a wider range of sexual behavior than is generally accepted.

The primary counselor first must assess the person's fears and feelings about sexuality, then be prepared to give information and support over a considerable period. While some people may be too shy for any but individual counseling, group process is often the most useful approach in the supportive phase of the therapy. In a group, people can gain strength as they find out that their own situation is not unique. The counselor aids group process by furnishing information, facilitating interaction, and supporting individuals when they need it.

The counselor should take a generally hopeful stance. Patients ordinarily come to the sessions with many fears, so if a counselor is overly fearful about creating false optimism, he or she may reinforce a patient's lack of confidence about the primary problem—acquiring a sex partner. When counselors fail to stress the positive aspects of sexuality, patients question even more strongly their ability to perform, become apathetic, and do not pursue a relationship. Hohmann's advise strikes us as sound:

In general, the cord-injured person should be encouraged to engage in whatever types of sexual activities are physiologically possible, pleasing, esthetic, gratifying, and acceptable to him and his partner. The counselor should begin by assuming that some genital functioning is possible until experience, time, and careful neurological examination demonstrate the contrary.(8)

The counselor should encourage the client's efforts to establish the human relationships that could lead to sexual relationships. Some adults who have been disabled all or most of their lives may never have had any sexual encounters or even any dates. They may well need support to achieve even a simple friendship with a member of the opposite sex. Discussion of the processes by which human relationships are formed and nourished may be a necessary part of the therapeutic process.

A progressive sequence of events must occur for two people to develop a satisfying sexual relationship. While nondisabled people also move through this process, they have the luxury of not noticing the steps and can believe that their sexual experiences were all beautifully spontaneous. The physically disabled are confronted by barriers that can interrupt each stage and make the whole process seem contrived. The four stages of this process are locating a possible mate, introducing oneself, establishing communication, and preparing for the sex act.

FINDING A PARTNER

Finding the possible partner—the basic step—is the first barrier for the physically disabled. Many withdraw from public life and are supported in their withdrawal by protective family members as well as the expectations of society. The disabled person fears the reactions of others to his deformity and his wheelchair. He is very conscious of the curiosity engendered by his appearance. It is important that the counselor help the client to see that the wheelchair, braces, or deformed limbs need not be deterrents to the development of friendly relationships.

Another reason for withdrawal is mobility itself. If one is confined to a wheelchair and cannot propel it, assistance from someone else is necessary. It is usually more difficult to approach someone of the opposite sex while a third party is standing by. A motorized chair, with specific adaptations for the condition of the occupant, is usually the answer to this problem. The more independent and socially active the disabled person is, the greater his or her probability for meeting someone of the opposite sex, or the same sex if that is the sexual preference.

The next stage, introduction, necessitates talking to the other person. The more severe the deformity, or the more difficulty one has with verbal communication, the more complex an introduction becomes. Because society has not fully accepted the idea of girls asking boys for dates, this step is even more difficult for women. The fact that many able-bodied people are apprehensive about approaching anyone in a wheelchair, and that many wheelchair occupants feel they are in an inferior position, may block any social interaction. If the disabled person does indeed want to start a relationship, he or she probably will have to open the conversation.

The disabled person has to be even more open verbally than is the norm for most people. In this regard, a counselor can help the client see that this more aggressive stance is called for.

After the disabled person has become acquainted with another person and wishes to pursue the relationship to a more profound level, fairly extensive communication usually must follow. At this stage, an able-bodied man can put his arm around a woman and both will know almost immediately, without many words, how the other feels. But a quadriplegic person, with limited or no movement in his upper extremities, must make all contacts verbally. This is where the barrier arises.

It is extremely difficult to ask a woman to put her arms around you and kiss you. The situation becomes even more complicated when the woman's cues are very subtle. The man is perplexed. How should he interpret those cues? He becomes even more reluctant to pursue the relationship. What is true for the man is even more true for the woman, and many potential relationships founder at this point.

PREPARATION

The last stage is preparation. For the disabled individual, sex cannot be as spontaneous as it can be for the able-bodied. Most quadriplegics must be lifted into bed, undressed, have their urinary apparatus removed, and their genital area washed. If the sexual companion is expected to do this, the request would have to be verbalized, and that would take extraordinary courage. There are alternatives. A relative, friend, or attendant can be asked to do these tasks, but this can create an awkward situation, and, if it is not managed carefully, the extra helper can depersonalize the relationship and embarrass all three.

If this entire process sounds planned, mechanical, and just not worth the effort, then our point has been well made. That is precisely the reason that a large number of physically disabled people never have a relationship that culminates in a sexual experience.

Once the disabled person has successfully participated in the sex act, the problem assumes lesser dimensions. Anxiety decreases and experimentation becomes possible. This experimentation may well include varying the position of the partners, oral-genital sex, the use of prostheses, or manual techniques for stimulation. There are a few reasonably good films available about these techniques.*

ATTITUDINAL BARRIERS

The counselor, bearing in mind that the technical barrier is less significant than the attitudinal one, must rember that many clients have grown up believing the masturbation would drive them insane or that the sex act should be performed only in the dark of night in the traditional positions. While the counselor should certainly try to avoid offending these

---

* Three films titled, "Just What Can You Do?" "Possibilities" and "Touching," are available from T. Coles, Multi Media Resource Center, #439 E. 340 Jones Street, San Francisco, California 94102.

sensibilities, he or she should at least give positive sanction to some experimentation.

Given the opportunity to participate, what are the probabilities for success in the sexual realm? For most people with muscular dystrophy, cerebral palsy, post-poliomyelitis damage, and similar disabling conditions, sexual performance is usually possible.

Patients with traumatic injuries to the spine face a more complex situation because the damage is often more serious and affects the four phases of the sexual cycle. These are excitation, plateau, orgasm, and resolution(9). Tumescence during excitation and the detumescence of the resolution phase are controlled by the autonomic nervous system, with innervation stemming primarily from the sacral portion of the cauda equina, and possibly through an ancillary pathway of innervation from the mid-thoracic region. Innervation for the plateau phase and consequent orgasm come primarily from the lumbar area(10).

Research done with patients who have spinal injuries suggests that, while sexual function is not certain, the picture is not nearly as gloomy as some people think. In a study of 529 men who had suffered damage to the spinal cord or cauda equina, Bors and Comarr found that 93 percent of those with complete upper motor neuron lesions were able to have erections. Patients whose lesions were not complete were, naturally, the most likely to be successful, but even those with complete transections of the cord were not impotent, particularly if their lesions were high. This is because tumescence and detumescence are possible as reflex processes without control of higher centers. Orgasm and ejaculation with complete lesions is much more problematic. Only 4 percent of patients with complete upper motor lesions and 18 percent of those with complete lower motor neuron lesions reported ejaculation(11).

Buttman indicates that there is a general agreement in the literature that between 52 and 94 percent of men with spinal injuries can have erections, 3 to 19.7 percent can ejaculate, and 6 to 14 percent can experience orgasm(12). Because of difficulty with ejaculation, only about 1 to 5 percent of men in various studies have sired children after their injury(13).

Comarr's study of 25 women disclosed that about half had irregular menstruation following their injuries, but that 23 eventually regained their menstrual function. Four of the 25 were pregnant when they were injured and five conceived after their injury. All nine delivered normal infants, eight of them vaginally. The one significant problem reported was a high incidence of pyelonephritis during and following pregnancy(14).

Few researchers have interviewed women patients regarding sexual activity after spinal cord injury. This dispartiy relative to men might be attributed to several factors. Since wars and sports activities are the major causes of cord injuries, fewer women have suffered this type of trauma. Moreover, women with cord damage are able to participate reasonably well in the sex act in the traditionally more passive role, so have seemed to have fewer problems. Also, women probably were less willing to discuss their problems with male researchers.

Both men and women whose lesions are complete have no sensation below the level of the injury, which naturally decreases subjective pleasures of sex. Nevertheless, most of the people we interviewed as well as those reported to the literature indicated that general bodily responses and stimulation above their injury are satisfying. The more significant satisfaction is probably not the physiological one, but the satisfaction of participating, albeit on a limited scale, in what is often considered to be the most significant social experience.

SECONDARY SEX COUNSELING

We assume that a clinical nurse specialist or nurse practioner might serve as a primary sex counselor. Nurses can make significant contributions as secondary sex counselors who are available to answer questions and listen to patients' concerns. Some patients, including shy women, seek out the female nurse for advice. But if they are given the "ask your doctor" answer they may conclude that their question was improper and never ask anyone. A nurse who is knowledgeable and comfortable discussing sex with the patient can help him or her and guide the patient to seek further help from the specialized sex counselor.

There are, of course, certain dangers involved in primary or secondary sex counseling. Because the subject is so intimate the patient may become emotionally involved with the counselor. Disabled persons, during their period of rehabilitation, need emotional support and a feeling of security. Therefore, anyone who shows a direct interest in their intimate problems may become a target for their feelings. This situation must be guarded and handled with the greatest care to prevent serious emotional damage to the patient, and to the counselor.

It is important to honestly let the patient know early that the relationship is a professional rather than a personal one. The nurse can make it clear that she or he is off limits sexually. The bond between the nurse counselor and client should be characterized by interest, concern, and shared problem solving. To reinforce this stance, conversations about persons who are real or potential love objects should always be focused outside the nurse-patient dyad.

Experienced nurse psychotherapists also advise that anyone who does counseling should have a consultant available to them. The consultant can be a colleague or an outside therapist whose role is to listen, give advice, and help the counselor regain perspective when problems develop. Hopefully, the counseling will help people who are disabled and fewer of them will be sentenced to a life without a loving sexual relationship.

REFERENCES

1. BORS, ERNEST, AND COMARR, A. E. Neurological disturbances of sexual function with special reference to 529 patients with spinal cord injury. *Urol.Survey* 10:191-222, Dec. 1960.
2. WEISS, A. J., AND DIAMOND, M. D. Sexual adjustment, identification, and attitudes of patients with myelopathy. *Arch.Phys.Med.* 47:245-250. Apr. 1966.
3. RIGHT to have sex—response to demands by spine-injured G. I.s. *Psychol.Today* 6:135-136. Oct, 1972.
4. SEX and the paraplegic. *Med.World News*, Jan. 14, 1972.
5. COMARR, A. E. Sex among patients with spinal cord and/or cauda equina injuries. *Med.Aspects Human Sexual.* 7:222-238, Mar. 1973.
6. RUGE, DANIEL. *Spinal Cord Injuries*. Springfield, Ill., Charles C Thomas, 1969, p. 51
7. WEISS AND DIAMOND. *op.cit.* p. 248.
8. HOHMANN, G. W. Considerations in the management of psychosexual readjustment in the cord injured male. *Rehab.Psychol.* 19(2):50-58. Summer 1972.
9. MASTERS, W. H., AND JOHNSON, V. E. *Human Sexual Response*. Boston. Little, Brown and Co., 1966.
10. RUSK, HOWARD, AND OTHERS. Roundtable: sex problem in paraplegia. *Med.Aspects Human Sexual.* 1:46-50. Dec. 1967.
11. BORS AND COMARR, *op.cit.*, p. 216.
12. GUTTMAN, SIR LUDWIG. *Spinal Cord Injuries: Comprehensive Management and Research*. Oxford. Blackwell Scientific Publications, 1973. pp. 446-478.
13. BORS AND COMARR. *op.cit.*, p. 216.
14. COMARR, A. E. Interesting observations on females with spinal cord injury. *Med.Serv.J.* (Canada) 22:651-661, July-Aug. 1966.

Janie Remembered

MATTIE TOLLEY

A victim of a car accident, Janie's screams were unintelligible. But students sensed that she was trying to communicate and patiently helped her accomplish a miracle.

"Janie, age 16, post car accident, neurological damage of undertermined degree," read my assignment, a cold introduction to one of my most valuable learning experiences as a student nurse. Janie had been riding with friends; her best friend was thrown through the windshield and killed instantly. Now, several days later, Janie had been transferred from the intensive care unit to the neurological floor and I was assigned to care for her.

A pretty girl, arms and legs held in splints to straighten contractures, Janie's only communication was an almost maddening, steady, high-pitched scream. Struggling to cope with her physical needs, I noted small behavior patterns. The pitch and loudness of her continual scream varied with her degree of comfort: louder when I manipulated her contracted limbs, quieter as I massaged her back, and finally ceasing as she sucked on small ice chips, the only nourishment that she accepted willingly. Her eyes followed my movements and turned to the door when anyone approached. Every now and then Janie's eyes suddenly looked terror stricken, and her screams echoed down the hallway. Janie could see and hear, but what did her mind tell her? What caused the unmistakable terror?

As a student, my observations were finer than my ability to interpret them. I consulted Janie's doctor. He was less than optimistic: irreversible

MS. TOLLEY *is a graduate of Hillcrest Medical Center School of Nursing, Tulsa, Okla. She has worked as a medical-surgical nurse and in relief and rehabilitation for Church World Service in Nigeria.*

brain damage, "vegetable," no progress expected, transfer soon to the state children's mental hospital, prepare mother. Listening staff nurses nodded wisely; already Janie had become the ward's most unpopular patient. Physically hard to handle and emotionally infuriating, she was a custodial case to be tolerated only as long as necessary.

But I continued to see minute improvements. Janie could be quieted by gentle chatter, back massage, caressing her cheek. There were foods she would eat without a murmur, others which she resisted. Was she trying to tell me what foods she liked and disliked? Janie puzzled me, but I could not dismiss her as a "vegetable." Her eyes spoke intelligently, sometimes with the fires of anger and fear, other times with gentle peace and joy. I checked out my observations with staff nurses. Sympathy I got: "Yes, it's hard to accept." Listened to I was not. My frustration grew. The doctor made token calls, stayed minutes only, perhaps because Janie started screaming the moment he opened the door. With what pain did she associate him?

As days passed, Janie's care was rotated among the students in our group. At last I had allies. Other students sensed intelligent responses in our patient. And Janie made clear that she had favorites. For those unfortunates she did not want caring for her, the day was a torturing, shrill scream. Many times one of the three students she preferred would be called, and the screams would quiet the moment we walked in, ceasing as we talked gently to her. Janie *could* communicate her needs and desires. We were sure. A cold war between staff and students was on. We would prove them wrong!

Perhaps our instructor was not as certain, but Janie was a beautiful educationer. Our outside reading doubled as ideas and concepts were explored, discussed, and compared to Janie. Our observation techniques were sharpened, compared, questioned. Our instructor stood by and let us think and try.

Janie was moved to a remote section of the ward. By day she was left totally to the students. The few days we had been promised stretched to weeks. Had we reached the doctor after all? We tried everything. Had Janie seen her friend killed? Did memories of the accident bring on the hideous cries, the terror? Was this traumatic regression?

I remembered a case study I had read about a regressed patient who was treated by handling him as a baby and slowly helping him to his real age level. When Janie was terrified, I held her close and rocked her. Slowly her tense body relaxed and the screaming ceased. It seemed to work. We tried it again, and again her body relaxed, her limbs straightened. Eventually she no longer screamed when students were on duty, nor did her arms and legs contract. The splints were discarded.

Much of the brain is unused, making it possible, sometimes, to train other cells to take on the functions of damaged or destroyed tissue. Could Janie be retrained? We consulted the physical therapist and tried it. Simple things first: sucking, chewing. Demonstration, repetition, encouragement. One day she took her milk through a straw. Another day she chewed solid food. Each feat was celebrated as a minor miracle, and we did not hide our joy from Janie, who quietly glowed. Speech. A baby's first word, "mama." Again repetition, encouragement. Ms. C. could not contain her joy the day Janie greeted her as "mama." Movement. "Squeeze my hand." She did. The doctor called in the physical therapist himself. We had a compassionate ally.

Slowly, Janie began to speak. First words, then phrases, then the magic sentence. "I want a hamburger." We laughed and cried with her mother. Janie got one hamburger STAT! The nursing staff was shocked. "A miracle, Janie is suddenly talking." We knew "suddenly" had been a long trudge toward this day.

It was the beginning for Janie. A few weeks later she was transferred, not to a mental facility but to a rehabilitation center to learn to walk again. Six months later our student group visited the rehabilitation center and asked for Janie. Our guide glowed. Janie was everyone's pride. Studying with a special tutor, improving daily, she could crawl now and would walk one day. Her intelligence? Unimpaired.

Did Janie remember us? She assured us she did. She remembered the caresses, the comforting words, being taught to chew, to grasp. And yes, she remembered the accident. I realized I had been right about the terror, the screams. As I hugged Janie a last goodbye, I made a silent vow to remember the slow miracle that had changed a "vegetable" into this vibrant, courageous girl.

Section V   Cerebral Vascular Disease: Acute Care and Rehabilitation

Stroke can be prevented by encouraging those persons who have experienced transient neurological deficits or who are hypertensive to seek medical care. If stroke occurs, immediate intervention is planned to prevent complications. The final articles in this section consider the multiple problems—motor, sensory, communication, and emotional—which demand the nurse's attention during the stroke victim's convalescence and rehabilitation.

Transient Ischemic Attacks

MARGARET R. KELLER • B. LIONEL TRUSCOTT

Nurses can help prevent strokes by encouraging people who experience short-lived neurological deficits to get prompt medical attention.

"I had such a pleasant swim, that last day of my vacation. I walked to my car and when I started to open the door I realized that my left hand and arm were numb. I managed to get the door open, the keys out of my purse and the ignition started, but had no "feel" of the steering wheel in my left hand. Then the feeling in my arm and hand gradually returned, and by the time I was out of the parking lot everything was fine. It never occurred to me that I needed medical attention."

The nurse who related this incident is now under medical care with a diagnosis of transient ischemic attack (TIA). When a second episode occurred that made the entire left side of her body feel "numb and useless," she sought medical advice.

Her history is typical of many patients with TIA. Nurses working on medical units in acute hospitals admit patients for observation who appear paralyzed on one side, have slurred speech, and, usually, normal vital signs. These patients appear to be well again within 24 hours, have no complaints, and are discharged in a few days. Nurses are often sur-

---

MS. KELLER *was nurse education coordinator of the Comprehensive Stroke Program of the North Carolina Comprehensive Regional Medical Program, and assistant professor of public health at Bowman Gray School of Medicine, Winston-Salem, N.C. at the time this paper was written. A graduate of Columbia Hospital School of Nursing, Wilkinsburg, Pa., she received a B.S. from the University of Pittsburgh, and a M.P.H. from the University of North Carolina at Chapel Hill.* DR. TRUSCOTT *is director of the North Carolina Comprehensive Stroke Program, and professor of neurology at Bowman Gray School of Medicine. He holds Ph.D. and M.D. degrees from Yale University, New Haven, Conn.*

prised when these same patients return six months or a year later with completed strokes and irreversible damage. Nurses in industry, public health, or nursing homes may also hear patients describing symptoms of transient ischemic attacks and not recognize that these patients should be referred for medical evaluation and treatment.

What is a transient ischemic attack? How does it differ from a "little stroke," or a vasospasm of cerebral arteries? "A focal cerebral ischemia of less than 24 hours duration" is perhaps the most concise description of this condition(1).

A transient ischemic attack is produced by a temporary reduction or loss of blood supply to a region of the brain, due to partial or total obstruction of an artery in the carotid or vertebrobasilar system, or to a critical fall in blood pressure. The most common obstruction is an embolus arising from an ulcerated plaque, for example, in the cervical carotid, or from a prosthetic heart valve, or a diseased heart valve during an episode of auricular fibrillation. In a person with widespread cerebrovascular disease, whose cerebral blood flow may be marginally adequate, sudden hypotension may precipitate an ischemic attack. Whatever the cause of TIA, blood supply is restored promptly and symptoms clear within 24 hours.

A transient ischemic attack may herald an impending stroke. Of 1,300 stroke patients identified by the North Carolina Comprehensive Stroke Program, six percent had experienced at least one TIA before developing a completed stroke. It is estimated that over a five year period 35 percent of patients with histories of TIA will have major strokes. In a city of 200,000 people, about 60 will experience TIAs each year, and over 20 of these will have strokes within the next five years(2).

DIAGNOSIS

In most cases the diagnosis can be made by determining whether the patient has had one or more of the following symptoms which cleared within 24 hours, and were not due to any other apparent cause, such as labyrinthitis, "sleeping on" a limb, and so on:
- Weakness or numbness of one side of the body
- Slurring, thickness, or loss of speech
- Blindness in one eye
- Double vision
- Sudden falls due to weakness of the legs
- Staggering or incoordinated walking
- Sudden movement or whirling of surrounding objects.

Because the signs of a TIA are short lived, it is rarely possible to con-

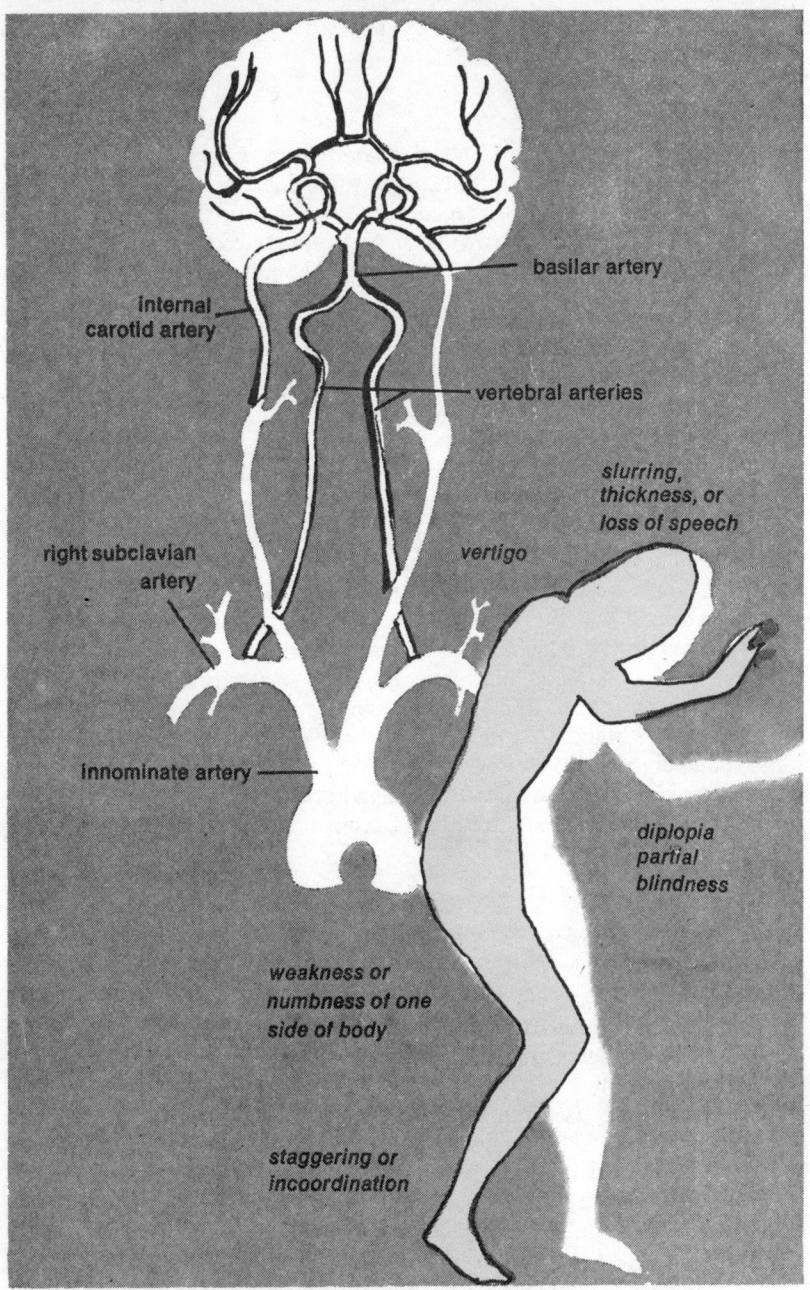

The carotid and vertebrobasilar arteries are the most frequent sites of obstruction in TIA, causing a variety of short-lived symptoms.

firm the diagnosis by neurological examination. Other signs, however, may indicate the presence of pathology sufficient to produce a TIA. Possible sources of emboli are revealed by a harsh bruit in the neck (suggesting the existence of narrowing or of an ulcerated plaque in the carotid), a prosthetic heart valve, or stenosis of the mitral valve and episodes of auricular fibrillation. Similarly, cholesterol or platelet fibrin emboli may be seen in retinal arterioles, indicating that the source of these clots may be an ulcerated plaque in a major vessel.

Certain other evidence may support the clinical impression that the patient has had a TIA and is stroke prone: elevated blood pressure, elevated fasting blood sugar, and abnormal Q wave or ST segment on the electrocardiogram(3). Increased serum cholesterol in patients below 50 years of age is also suggestive(4). Definitive evidence is obtained if an angiogram shows an area of stenosis or ulcerated plaque.

Although several neurological disorders may mimic a TIA, the differential diagnosis is rarely difficult. The transient blurring of vision, numbness, and ataxia which many patients with multiple sclerosis experience usually occur in their teens or twenties, and may persist for days or for the rest of the patient's life. A completed stroke is differentiated by weakness or numbness, loss of speech, and other symptoms which persist longer than 24 hours. A tumor or subdural hematoma produces symptoms relatively slowly, causes progressive worsening of the neurological deficit, and is preceded by headache, head injury, or personality changes. An abnormal lumbar puncture, brain scan, or angiogram will clinch the diagnosis.

TREATMENT

Heparin or coumadin (Warfarin) may be given if the cause of the TIA is an embolus and there is no surgically correctable or accessible source of emboli, or the patient's physical status precludes surgery. Major contraindications to anticoagulation are hypertension, gastric or urinary bladder ulcers, lack of laboratory facilities, or inability of the patient to cooperate.

Vascular surgery is often indicated to reduce the frequency of TIAs and prevent stroke. The lesions most accessible to surgery are located in the cervical carotid artery or arch of the aorta, where plaques can be removed by endarterectomy, or in narrowed vessel segments which can be by-passed by vein grafts or Dacron prostheses.

Prompt identification and treatment of patients with hypertension and transient ischemic attacks would constitute a major step toward stroke prevention. Because of her early and frequent contact with patients, the nurse can help identify the patient with TIA and advise him to see a physician. Wherever nurses work, they should recognize the possible implication of transient symptoms described by a person who does not believe they are sufficiently important to bring to a doctor's attention. By assessing the patient's reported symptoms, a nurse can very quickly determine whether medical evaluation is necessary. These few minutes spent by the nurse may help shape his future.

REFERENCES

1. WHISNANT, J. P., AND OTHERS. Natural history of stroke in Rochester, Minnesota. 1945 through 1954. *Stroke* 2:12 Jan.-Feb. 1971.
2. GOLDENER, J. C., AND OTHERS. Long-term prognosis of transient cerebral ischemic attacks. *Stroke* 2:160-167, Mar.-Apr. 1971.
3. JOINT COMMITTEE FOR STROKE FACILITIES, CLINICAL PREVENTION OF STROKE. *Guidelines.* (To be published)
4. KANNEL, W. B. Current status of the epidemiology of brain infarction associated with occlusive arterial disease. *Stroke* 2:295-318, July-Aug. 1971.

Stroke

ANN M. JACOBANSKY

Prevention of further deterioration is a key goal in the nursing care of these patients.

When the term "stroke" is used, it usually connotes a symptom or a group of symptoms related to faulty functioning of the brain. This process can result in impaired vital functions (heart and respiratory mechanisms) and such focal neurologic signs and symptoms as headache, nausea and vomiting, visual disturbances, paresis, paralysis, aphasia, seizures, and cranial nerve palsies. Clinical signs and symptoms vary depending on the location and size of the lesion caused by an interruption in cerebral blood flow.

Perhaps the term, cerebrovascular accident (CVA), which is synonymous with stroke, more clearly defines the emergency nature of this illness. Its onset is usually quite abrupt, as the blood supply to a part of the brain is suddenly interrupted by a thrombotic occlusion in or hemorrhage from a cerebral artery. The acute phase is usually considered to be the first 24 to 48 hours following the ictus, but it can extend to many days and weeks. Symptoms and the patient's general condition can change rapidly during the acute phase. And, no matter how minor the symptoms may initially appear, these patients are often quite seriously ill.

For example, Ms. N.M., a 61-year-old woman, was admitted by ambulance to the emergency room. Two days prior to admission, she had become drowsy and complained of weakness in her upper and lower left extremities. She was somnolent but conscious on admission and had a left hemiplegia. Her somnolence increased and by the third day she was

> MS. JACOBANSKY *is a professor of nursing at Duke University School of Nursing in Durham, N.C. She was graduated from Shadyside Hospital School of Nursing in Pittsburgh, Pa., and received her B.S.N. and her M.Ed. degrees from the University of Pittsburgh.*

in a deep coma. Her respirations became increasingly irregular and stertorous. Muscle spasms of her left side were noted periodically. She never regained consciousness and she died on the 27th day of hospitalization.

Like Ms. N.M., the majority of CVA patients do not present in coma. The patient may be alert, lethargic, somnolent, stuporous, or comatosed. He may be completely oriented or disoriented. His judgment may be sound or impaired. He may be emotionally labile. His level of consciousness may change over a period of hours or days from alertness to coma, or vice versa. "The depth and duration of coma are diagnostically significant; the shorter and less deep the coma, the better the prognosis"(1).

An assessment of the level of consciousness is extremely important in identifying and preventing further deterioration and in determining the patient's capability of meeting his own needs. The needs of an acutely ill CVA patient are not unlike those of other acutely ill patients: rest and safety, patent airway, elimination (bladder and bowel), positioning, skin care, mouth care, nutrition, communication and observation (vital signs, skin integrity, and sensory and motor signs).

REST AND SAFETY

Neurologists advocate bedrest for all patients presenting signs or symptoms of a CVA. Unless another position is specified or indicated by such conditions as breathing difficulty or cardiac failure, a flat position without a pillow for 24 to 36 hours is often preferred to assure an adequate cerebral blood flow(2). But bedrest means more than keeping the patient in bed; it is interpreted to mean doing for the patient everything he would normally do for himself to avoid increasing intravascular pressure during the acute phase(3). Also, during this period, patients should not be transported unnecessarily for such diagnostic tests as x-ray and electrocardiogram, which can be done at the bedside.

For CVA patients exhibiting restlessness, sedatives or tranquilizers may be prescribed. But, because such drugs may make it difficult to accurately assess a patient's level of consciousness, other measures to decrease restlessness ought to be tried first. The presence of family members may have a soothing effect on some restless patients. By brushing or combing the patient's hair, sponging his face and hands, or merely holding the unaffected hand, the family may be able to relax the patient. While the patient is on bedrest, family members may share in his care; this may help both the patient and the family. Family members and visitors need to be made aware of the patient's neurologic deficits and must be cautioned about prodding or pressuring the aphasic patient to speak or the hemiplegic patient to move his paralyzed limbs.

Siderails provide some degree of safety for these patients. Occasionally, it is advisable to use such other precautionary measures as restraints, particularly for disoriented or forgetful patients when they are unattended. A vest restraint is usually adequate. If a patient appears quiet and relaxed with visitors, siderails and restraints may be removed if the visitors are instructed in the importance and use of these safety aids.

MAINTENANCE OF PATENT AIRWAY

All patients, other than those presenting in coma, should be instructed to deep breathe and cough and to change position as frequently as possible. Family members can be instructed in the importance of this, and, during their visits, they can remind the patient and assist him in turning.

Frequent turning and positioning, along with deep breathing and coughing exercises are sufficient for most patients. But, patients who have a decreased level of consciousness (somnolence, stupor, or coma), dysarthria, shallow breathing, or an inability to deep cough are likely to need assistance in maintaining and supporting respiratory function. These patients may accumulate bronchial secretions, which tend to reduce ventilation and can lead to serious complications. To improve pulmonary ventilation, some patients may require nasopharyngeal suctioning, oxygen administration, intermittent positive pressure breathing exercises, or some combination of these measures.

Constant surveillance is essential to determine whether a patient is maintaining ventilation adequate for his needs without assistance or whether assistive measures must be instituted. For the patient unable to breathe or cough deeply, intermittent positive pressure breathing exercises may be helpful. Oxygen therapy is useful for a patient unable to breathe or cough deeply, intermittent positive pressure breathing exercises may be helpful. Oxygen therapy is useful for a patient with diminished cardiac output or respiratory exchange. A side-lying position, on a level bed, with the head slightly extended, facilitates deep breathing. For the comatosed patient, this position helps to prevent aspiration of secretions and keeps the tongue from obstructing the pharynx. An oral airway may also be ordered to keep the tongue in place and the airway patent. And, for some patients, a tracheostomy may be performed to reduce the respiratory dead space and facilitate tracheobronchial cleansing(4).

POSITIONING

All comatose, stuporous, and somnolent patients need to be positioned in proper body alignment and this position needs to be changed frequently. This is important for adequate ventilation, to relieve pressure from certain skin areas, and to prevent deformities.

A prone or three-quarter prone position is physiologically desirable, and in these positions, the patient is less likely to move automatically into a poor supine position. However, they are rarely used because patients tend to display fear or apprehension in these positions.

An optimal position for the hemiplegic patient is with the upper extremities abducted and externally rotated to protect the shoulder from becoming contracted; the hand slightly higher than the forearm and shoulder to prevent edema; the leg in a neutral position, that is, neither internally nor externally rotated; and the foot at a right angle to the leg. With loss of proprioception, the stronger "pulling" muscles will pull the fingers, wrist, elbow, knee and hip into "flexed" positions. Thus, one of the first nursing considerations is the prevention of additional deformities in the paralyzed hand, arm, foot, and leg.

If attention is not given to proper positioning for protection of muscle and joint functioning early, it is likely that the patient will develop deformities which can be seriously handicapping; these include: "adduction and internal rotation at the hip; knee and plantar flexion; and ankle inversion"(5).

Positioning is a supportive as well as preventive nursing measure; supportive in terms of musculo-skeletal and respiratory functions; preventive in terms of contractures and deformities, disuse muscular weaknesses, pneumonia or atelectasis, and skin breakdown. Proper positioning involves changing the patient's position at least every two hours. The bed should be kept as flat as tolerated to prevent hip flexion, compromised chest expansion due to slumping, and skin irritation resulting from the friction of sliding down in bed.

NUTRITION

During the first 24 to 48 hours following the ictus, intravenous fluids are usually administered according to the patient's nutritional needs, including the need for adjustment of the electrolyte balance. If the patient is unconscious, stuporous, or unable to swallow, fluids are normally administered by nasogastric tube after the second or third day.

In addition to water, tube feedings which consist of a liquid formula of nutrients (proteins, fats, carbohydrates, minerals, and vitamins) must be supplied in suitable amounts if adequate nutrition is to be assured. The formula and water feedings are ordered on a regular schedule of 2 to 4 hour intervals for a total of 2,000 to 3,000 cc. in a 24-hour period. Feedings may be ordered as a continuous drip for a period of 8 to 12 hours.

If the patient shows signs of consciousness, ice chips in small amounts may be used to test swallowing ability. If the swallowing mechanism is functioning, water and fluids by mouth are then attempted. Patients with facial paralysis may have difficulty trying to drink through a straw and may do better drinking from a cup. Patients with dysphagia may continue to exhibit some difficulty in swallowing; in progressing these patients from oral liquids to solid food, caution must be exercised in testing with water since aspiration may result. Some patients who can tolerate ice chips, but not liquids, may have less difficulty with such semi-soft foods as gelatin. For the patient who has no problem swallowing but difficulty in drinking from a cup or a straw, a training cup or rubber tipped syringe may be used.

Unless otherwise ordered, the 24-hour fluid intake should total 2,000 to 3,000 cc. To ensure an adequate fluid balance, accurate intake and output records are of prime importance.

As patients are able to tolerate solid food, assistance with feeding should be available. The patient may need help in cutting his food into bite size pieces, or food may have to be placed within his vision and reach to facilitate self-feeding.

Most right-handed patients with right hemiplegia experience difficulty in moving the food to their mouths with their left hands. Spilling and sloppiness are common, particularly early in the experience. A bath towel serves well to catch food and liquids and to protect clothing. Patients who present facial and one-side-of-tongue weakness will encounter difficulty in pushing a bolus of food to the back of the mouth. The bolus may remain in the affected cheek until removed.

Nausea and vomiting are not common, but a poor appetite is. For most patients, fluids have to be encouraged and offered frequently. Some patients will do well when fluids or food are offered, but will rarely ask for nourishment or water. Family members need to be instructed about encouraging fluids and need to be encouraged to help in feeding when feasible. Food or fluid likes or dislikes are rarely expressed; however, preferred foods are more likely to be accepted and with greater relish than those foods routinely supplied.

ELIMINATION

Urinary incontinence is a rather common problem with these patients. Micturition is both voluntary and involuntary. The voluntary portion is controlled by a portion of the brain and the involuntary by reflex act of spinal nerves. Thus, when the brain control is affected, as in stroke, the bladder may empty when increased intra-bladder pressure stimulates the spinal nerve reflex. For these patients, the awareness of the urge to void and the automatic reflex act tend to be almost simultaneous. Unless provision is made for voluntary emptying of the bladder immediately on the urge to void, involuntary emptying will occur.

External or condom catheters are used for most male patients and indwelling Foley catheters for female patients. Except for patients whose urine must be tested frequently (diabetics), catheter insertion for incontinence may be delayed for the first 24 hours in order to determine the nature of urinary incontinence and whether an indwelling catheter is the only alternative for the good of the patient. Sometimes, placing the patient on a bed pan at regular intervals and setting up a voiding schedule will make catheterization and all its risks unnecessary.

In bowel elimination, constipation may be more common than bowel incontinence. When for some reason, the fecal material is slowed down in its passage through the colon, as in the CVA patient on bedrest, water continues to be absorbed by the absorption surfaces making the fecal material more solid as it enters the rectum—the result is constipation and ultimately impaction. Thus, admission orders ought to include stool softeners and laxatives, either on a regular schedule or as needed. For most patients, the combination of a laxative and a stool softener will be sufficient. However, suppositories or enemas may also be required to establish bowel habits. Then, when waste products do enter the rectum, reflexes passing between the rectum and spinal cord may cause automatic emptying of the rectum when it becomes full. These rectal reflexes are normally inhibited by portions of the brain until an opportune time for evacuation; but when the state of consciousness is affected or when there is damage in the controlling portions of the brain, automatic emptying or incontinence can result.

COMMUNICATION

Following a CVA, some patients are able to express their needs. However, many patients are not. This can be due to coma, confusion and disorientation, or aphasia. Of these, aphasia probably is the most distressing for the patient, his family, and nursing personnel.

Some patients with sensory aphasia can follow simple verbal commands with relative ease, some can follow verbal commands accompanied by gestures. But, some are unable to follow even such simple, one-word-and-a-gesture commands as a nurse pointing first to her open mouth and then to the patient's mouth while saying, "open."

Patients with motor aphasia may attempt speech even though garbled or may be either unable or unwilling to express any sound. These patients often gesticulate—pointing, nodding, or shaking their heads, using pantomime, and then smiling and vigorously nodding their heads when gestures are correctly interpreted.

A major human need is the ability to express self with words and language. For the aphasic patient, a sequel of his brain damage is interference with his language system. The messages communicated to him may be distorted, may be only partially interpreted, or not interpreted at all; in trying to send messages, the patient may have trouble with word formulation and production. Such communication problems can cause the patient, his family, and the staff to become frustrated. Some patients then resign themselves to the problem; others persist with great patience in attempting to communicate.

Knowing the location of damage can help a nurse determine what she can expect from a patient. If a right-handed patient has right hemiplegia, the damage is probably in his dominant (left) cerebral hemisphere; if he has left hemiplegia, the damage is probably in his minor (right) cerebral hemisphere. Damage to the left cerebral hemisphere most often results in verbal deficits, whereas damage to the right cerebral hemisphere usually results in visual or auditory deficits, such as homonymous hemianopia in which the patient loses half of his field of vision in each eye(6). Some areas of the language system may be more affected than others; but if there is difficulty in one, there usually is some difficulty in all areas.

In communicating with the aphasic patient, attention needs to be given to increasing the number and variety of auditory and visual stimuli and to allowing time for the patient to respond if a response is expected. Other means which may promote communication include speaking directly to the patient—looking at him and having him look at the speaker—and using simple one-word commands and gestures. Sometimes, transmission of words is facilitated by speaking in a normal tone of voice, but more slowly than usual. Some loss in transmission may be prevented by keeping the sentence structure simple and brief; by relying on nouns and verbs; by eliminating unnecessary conjunctions, prepositions, adjectives, and so forth, and by repeating key words.

CONCLUSION

Although most of the patients who survive a stroke cannot be "cured," many can be helped to perform at least the simple activities of daily living. Patients who seem most critical can often improve dramatically with intensive nursing care during the acute phase. And, by including the family in the patient's care, improvement may continue after discharge.

For example, 56-year-old Ms. W. had collapsed at home and was brought by ambulance to the emergency room. On admission, she was comatosed, cyanotic, and the right side of her face sagged. She was placed in an oxygen tent. Within eight hours, she began to respond slightly to deep pressure on the left side. She then became extremely restless after 12 hours and right hemiplegia was noted. Aphasia was noted as she regained consciousness. Finally, on the fourth day post ictus, Ms. W.'s restlessness decreased and some movement was noted in her extremities, but her aphasia persisted. Full movement of all limbs returned by the end of the first week. She was unable to follow verbal commands. However, she followed through on assistance in positioning and in getting out of bed. She was able to take fluids orally on the fifth day and progressed to feeding herself by the end of the first week. She walked unsupported on the eleventh day. Periodic bowel and bladder incontinence continued until discharge. Also, she used poor judgment in all activities, feeding, getting out of bed, and dressing. Her family (husband, daughter, or sister) stayed with her constantly and assisted with her care—encouraging use of the bathroom, assisting in feeding, and attempting communication. Her judgment remained questionable until the day of discharge, which was 19 days after admission. Ms. W. was discharged to home with provision for family and attendant care. Speech therapy was begun at home shortly after her discharge.

Ms. W. certainly was not "cured," but she continued to improve and her existence is far from vegetative.

REFERENCES

1. MILLER, M. B. Life history of the stroke syndrome. *J.Am.Geriatr. Soc.* 16:603-617, May 1968.
2. TYLER, H. R. Modern concepts of the pathogenesis, diagnosis and treatment of cerebrovascular accidents. *Med.Clin.North Am.* 44:1215-1236, Sept. 1960.
3. KIRGIS, H. D., AND OTHERS. Strokes and their treatment. *Geriatrics* 23:144-159, Feb. 1968.
4. MCHENRY, I. C., JR., AND JAFFE, M. E. Cerebrovascular disease. Part 2. Management, *GP* 37:98-106, Apr. 1968.
5. NOVAK, JOSEPH. Rehabilitation of the hemiplegic patient. *Pa.Med. J.* 68:43-46, Mar.
6. *Ibid.*

BIBLIOGRAPHY

GORDON, E. E. Early application of physical medicine to stroke. *J.Rehabil.* 29:26-29, Nov.-Dec. 1963.

KURTZKE, J. L. *Epidemiology of Cerebrovascular Disease.* New York, Springer-Verlag, 1969.

SCHAAFSMA, S. On the differential diagnosis between cerebral hemorrhage and infarction. *J.Neurol.Sci.* 7:83-95, July-Aug. 1968.

TOOLE, J. F., AND PATEL, A. N. *Cerebrovascular Disorders.* New York, McGraw-Hill Book Co., 1967, pp. 569-577.

Subarachnoid Hemorrhage

MARJORIE MADDOX

> *Increased intracranial pressure, renewed bleeding, and the complications of prolonged bedrest are only a few of the problems that may arise.*

Ms. D., a 54-year-old woman, was brought to the emergency room by her family, who had found her unconscious. She had complained of a headache and, after taking two aspirin, had gone into the bedroom to lie down. Her family's attempts to arouse her later were unsuccessful. Bilateral carotid arteriograms completed before her admission to the neurosurgical unit showed a vertebral-artery aneurysm. Ms. D.'s condition indicated that the aneurysm was either leaking or had ruptured, and that she had sustained a subarachnoid hemorrhage.

By the time Ms. D. reached our unit, she was somnolent. Her blood pressure was high but her pupils were equal and reactive. Although her handgrips were strong bilaterally, she had some loss of motor function in her right leg. Because an intracranial hemorrhage occupies space in the cranial vault it raises intracranial pressure. This increases pressure on the optic nerve, which can impair vision. Therefore, Ms. D.'s difficulty in focusing was not unusual. Double vision may occur if the third, fourth, or sixth nerves are affected. Ptosis also may be present.

Ms. D. complained of a persistent, occipital headache. She also complained of pain when her head was tilted forward. Due to the sudden onset of her mental clouding and the severity of her headache, her vital and neurological signs were taken every 15 minutes to detect any signs of rising intracranial pressure.

Ms. D. had had mild, transient headaches all her life, but a persistent

---

MS. MADDOX *is a graduate of St. Luke's Hospital School of Nursing, St. Louis, Mo. She is a staff nurse on the neurosurgical unit at Duke University Medical Center, Durham, N.C.*

headache for the past few weeks. Often an initial, minor bleed goes undetected for some hours because the person believes his headache is a tension or migraine headache, takes aspirin, and lies down. If it is caused by cerebral bleeding, the headache is still present when the person wakes up. Because blood is irritating locally, symptoms of meningitis often accompany a hemorrhage and may mask the initial bleed. Because an aneurysm occupies space, its symptoms may be mistaken for those of a brain tumor.

A subarachnoid hemorrhage occurs when an aneurysm ruptures into the subarachnoid space. Aneurysms, which are sac-like dilatations of blood vessel walls, vary in size. Some are as tiny as a pea; others are the size of an orange. Larger aneurysms may erode skull bones. Most intracranial aneurysms are located near the basilar surface of the skull, and half of them arise from the internal carotid or the middle cerebral arteries. Aneurysms usually are found at the junction of main vessels, and 85 percent are in the circle of Willis. Usually the aneurysm is single, but occasionally they may be multiple. In persons who are 40 to 50 years old, the primary nontraumatic cause of intracranial hemorrhage is aneurysm(1).

Two tests are used to diagnose subarachnoid hemorrhage. A lumbar puncture is performed to obtain spinal fluid for cell count, protein levels, and culture. Usually the cerebrospinal fluid is grossly bloody and its opening pressure is elevated. Only the amount of spinal fluid needed for diagnostic testing is removed because a sudden and pronounced drop in spinal fluid pressure can precipitate renewed bleeding. Ms. D.'s first lumbar puncture was grossly bloody. Blood remains in the spinal fluid for four hours to 20 days after the initial bleed. Ms. D.'s spinal fluid was bloody for 10 days and then cleared.

Another definitive test is the carotid arteriogram. Radiopaque dye is injected into the carotid arteries to outline the cerebral circulatory system. With this test the site, size, and nature of pathological processes can be determined, and tumors, abscesses, aneurysms, or hematomas that grossly distort the normal vascular pattern can be localized. The test is contraindicated in the presence of severe liver, kidney, or thyroid disease. After an arteriogram, frequent vital and neurological signs should be taken. Because edema at the dye-injection site may cause airway obstruction, a tracheostomy tray is placed at the patient's bedside. An ice collar is applied to the patient's neck to control edema.

Ms. D.'s bleed was minor. Her care was directed toward the early recognition and prevention of complications and treatment of her primary neurological problem.

LEVELS OF CONSCIOUSNESS

LETHARGY	Patient's speech is slowed. He exhibits a delayed response to verbal suggestions.
SOMNOLENCE	Patient is excessively drowsy. He responds to verbal and tactile stimuli by mumbling or with jerking movements.
STUPOR	Patient reacts only to loud auditory or painful stimuli. He reacts by grimacing or withdrawing.
COMA	Patient does not react to auditory or painful stimuli.

Continued or recurrent bleeding from a ruptured or leaking aneurysm increases pressure on the cerebral contents, and 40 to 50 percent of patients with subarachnoid hemorrhage die within eight weeks after the initial bleed(1). Therefore, these patients must be observed closely for signs of increasing intracranial pressure. These signs should not be confused with those of shock. With increased intracranial hemorrhage the pulse slows to 40 or 50 and bounds. The pulse pressure widens. Whenever a rising blood pressure is observed in conjunction with a slowed pulse, increased intracranial pressure should be suspected. The patient's pupils should be inspected for equality and reactivity, and the equality and strength of his handgrips should be noted. Changes in the patient's level of consciousness may be the first indication that intracranial pressure is rising. Therefore, frequent checks of mentation are made.

Immediately after an intracranial bleed, measures are taken to prevent vomiting, straining, sneezing, coughing, and hiccoughing because these may increase intracranial pressure and stimulate more bleeding. The primary goals of nursing care are to prevent the complications of bedrest and the chances of a second bleed, which may prove fatal. The patient should receive minimal stimulation. Activity is restricted and visitors are limited. The environment must be kept quiet and the room semi-dark. The patient should remain flat in bed, but can turn from side to side. Vigorous suctioning and deep breathing exercises are avoided. Axillary temperatures are taken. Rectal temperature taking may stimulate the vagus nerve, and oral thermometers could prove hazardous if the patient seizes.

Codeine or aspirin is given to relieve the severe headache that accompanies hemorrhage. These drugs have a minimal depressant effect on the central nervous system—an important consideration in the care of persons with increased intracranial pressure. Antihypertensives may be given to lower the patient's blood pressure to normotensive or prehemorrhage levels. Diphenylhydantoin (Dilantin) and phenobarbital are used to control generalized seizures if they develop. Phenobarbital may also be given to sedate the patient and so prevent activity that may induce bleeding.

These patients often require a special bowel regimen to prevent constipation and straining. Stool softeners and cathartics are given. Enemas should not be given unless the patient has a fecal impaction. Then, oil retention enema followed by a cathartic is most effective.

Aminocaproic acid (Amicar) has been used experimentally in the treatment of subarachnoid hemorrhage. Amicar prevents rebleeding by inhibiting clot lysis throughout the body. Amicar crosses the blood-brain barrier and eliminates all measurable fibrinolytic activity in the spinal fluid. There is a high incidence of rebleeding 10 to 14 days following an initial subarachnoid hemorrhage. This is strikingly similar to the time required for the recanalization of thrombi in blood vessels. Therefore, it is possible that the fibrinolytic resolution of the thrombus in the aneurysm may cause rebleeding(2). The drug is contraindicated in patients with ischemic heart disease, renal insufficiency, or history of pulmonary embolism.

Because this treatment is experimental, a permit must be signed by the patient or his immediate family before treatment is begun. Blood tests, including a complete blood count, chemical profile, partial thromboplastin time (PTT), plasma fibrinogen levels, and a streptokinase clot lysis time, are done before administration begins, after one week of therapy, and again after two weeks. We use a solution of 288 cc. of dextrose 5% water plus 72 cc. (18 Gm.) of Amicar. This is administered intravenously over a 12-hour period, so that a total of 36 gms. is given each 24 hours. Patients do experience nausea and diarrhea as a result of this therapy, but these can be controlled(3).

Several methods of lowering intracranial pressure may be used. For patients who are hypertensive, fluids are limited to 800 to 1,200 cc./day. Saturated solution of magnesium sulfate may be given every morning, or hypertonic solution administered intravenously. Both solutions promote diuresis with consequent reduction of cerebral edema. An accurate record of intake and output is essential. Occasionally, spinal fluid is removed during a series of lumbar punctures in an attempt to lower intracranial pressure(4).

The presence of blood on the vessels acts as an irritant and causes significant vasospasm of the branches of the circle of Willis. Vasospasm may cause focal neurological deficits. Therefore, as the patient's condition stabilizes he must be watched continuously for any changes in ocular signs, vomiting, pain, convulsions, or motor or sensory deficits. Surgery is contraindicated as long as these vessels remain in spasm.

It is also important to consider the person's emotional status. Family members should be involved in aspects of his care so they can support him emotionally. Often, a good listener can help the patient work through the grieving which accompanies any serious and potentially fatal illness. However, family members often need reassurance and explanations before they can help the patient. Simple explanations of pertinent information about his condition are provided, and basic illustrations often help.

The necessary restriction on visitors should be explained and enforced tactfully. We provide a clip board outside the door so that visitors can leave messages. However, well-meaning visitors may not take "no" for an answer. Then, the seriousness of the situation and the hazards of overstimulating the patient must be explained bluntly.

Surgery is the treatment of choice to prevent recurrent bleeding in patients with subarachnoid hemorrhage from a ruptured aneurysm. However, surgery is delayed until the patient's condition has stabilized, usually in about two to six weeks.

The first week is the most critical period. Cerebral edema, blood clots, and vasospasm threaten the integrity of cerebral function, and there is the ever-present risk of bleeding. When this occurs, it is usually sudden and, if severe enough, fatal. Attempts at immediate surgical intervention usually are in vain. A grand mal seizure may herald an initial or subsequent severe bleed. Anticonvulsants usually are ineffective, and can mask the real problem if given in large and repeated dosages. If the patient does not respond to one dose of anticonvulsant drug, he should be observed for signs of increased intracranial pressure and measures should be instituted to correct it.

Ms. D. progressed well, without recurrence of bleeding or excessive vasospasm. Her blood pressure stabilized between 130/90 and 140/100 and her pupils remained equal and reactive. Her handgrips remained strong and equal. After two weeks of medical therapy, Ms. D. had a second arteriogram, which indicated that vasospasm had subsided and surgical repair was now possible.

The clipping of an aneurysm is a tense surgical procedure. The mortality associated with surgical repair of internal aneurysms is about 30 percent(2). Several procedures may be used. Clips are placed on either side of the aneurysm and it is clipped at the neck, or muscle may be wrapped around it. Aneurysms that cannot be repaired or clamped internally can be treated externally with a carotid, or Crutchfield, clamp.

Ms. D. had a suboccipital craniectomy. The vertebral-artery aneurysm was isolated and wrapped with fascia. After surgery, she returned to the intensive care area of our unit. Postoperatively, the patient is liable to develop any of the complications associated with surgery, especially thrombophlebitis. These patients also must be observed for any signs of periocular edema, hyperthermia, and speech disturbances. Changes in the patient's personality and behavior may be noted.

Ms. D.'s neurological and vital signs were taken frequently and she remained under very close observation. Her bed was elevated 30 degrees to increase the venous flow of blood. Her diet consisted of ice chips, then clear liquids, and then progressed to regular foods.

External occlusion of the carotid artery by a Crutchfield clamp is the treatment of choice for an aneurysm that cannot be reached surgically—for example, when it lies at the junction of many vessels and cannot be clipped without damaging them, or if the aneurysm is too massive, or if clipping has been unsuccessful. Progressive turns of the clamp cause it to occlude the carotid artery completely and thus block the blood supply to the aneurysm.

After the patient has been medicated for pain, the clamp is turned once daily by the surgeon. After each adjustment, frequent vital signs are taken to detect any untoward reaction to the decrease in carotid blood flow. Special precautions are taken to prevent accidental rotation or dislodging of the clamp. Limited activity is enforced. Sometimes a mild sedative is given to help the person relax and sleep. Communication is by written messages; very little talking is allowed. To discourage jaw movement, the patient receives intravenous fluids only. The clamp site must not be disturbed. A plastic cup may be taped lightly but securely over the site. Some patients must be restrained to remind them not to raise their arms and accidentally bump the clamp. After discharge, patients treated with the clamp must remain in bed at home for 30 days.

During the convalescent period, the patient's condition is evaluated constantly by each member of the health care team. Any residual disabilities are noted and rehabilitation is begun immediately. If he has been treated by intracranial surgery, the patient begins walking three or four days postoperatively.

A physical therapist helped Ms. D. with progressive ambulation. Eventually, she was using a walker and visiting with her family. Eight days after her operation, Ms. D.'s sutures were removed. After this, her head was washed with an antiseptic solution every morning for five days. Men wear skull caps and women wear bonnets or wigs.

Ms. D. was able to return home five weeks after her operation. She had no residual problems and did not bleed again.

Whether it is caused by a ruptured aneurysm or trauma, subarachnoid hemorrhage is a serious and frequently fatal condition. Excellent nursing care can minimize residual deficits by trying to prevent the recurrence of bleeding and the development of complications secondary to the necessarily prolonged inactivity that these patients experience.

REFERENCES

1. WALTON, J. N. *Essentials of Neurology*. 2d ed. Philadelphia, J. B. Lippincott Co., 1968, pp. 303-304.
2. PORTER, J. N., AND OTHERS. Fibrinolytic activity of the spinal fluid and meninges. *Surg. Forum* 27:427, 1966.
3. GIBBS, J. R., AND O'GORMAN, P. Fibrinolysis in subarachnoid haemorrhage. *Postgrad.Med.J.* 43:779-784, Dec. 1967.
4. DE GUTIERREZ-MAHONEY, C. G., AND CARNI, ESTA. *Neurological and Neurosurgical Nursing*. 4th ed. St. Louis, C. V. Mosby Co., 1965.

Motor Skill Rehabilitation for Hemiplegic Patients

MARJORIE PFAUDLER

Once past the acute phase of a stroke, the hemiplegic patient must relearn the simple activities of daily living. Planning and implementing this retraining requires knowledge of both the physical and behavioral sciences.

What is the fate of the men and women who were productive members of their families and communities until they suffered strokes? They can become completely dependent or, with truly professional care, can achieve a measure of independence and self-esteem.

Professional care requires the full and detailed use of the nursing process: assessment to determine problems, planning, implementation, and evaluation. In assessing the physical and psychosocial abilities and limitations of an individual and his family, all persons involved with his care will determine which problems they can handle best and plan accordingly. Whatever plans are made, the patient and his family must participate if the plan is to succeed. Plans must be changed as the status of the stroke patient changes.

The nurse is usually the long-term supportive professional who can lend consistency, coordination, and direction to the care plan. The nurse must take part in regular evaluation of the patient's progress to keep the plan appropriate, and must incorporate principles of teaching in providing care.

MS. PFAUDLER *is associate professor of nursing at the University of Rochester, N.Y. She has a B.S. degree from the University of Rochester and an M.A. degree from Teachers College, Columbia University, N.Y. This study was supported in part by USPHS grants NU00520-01, NU00250-02, and NU00520-03.*

ASSESSMENT CONSIDERATIONS

An individual with limited physical ability requires much greater energy expenditure from all body systems for his activities. Therefore, all persons working with such a patient must have accurate information about his cardiac status, general circulation, respiratory capacity, chronic medical problems, such as diabetes or arthritis, orthopedic problems, and any other limiting conditions. Without this information, the physical capacity of the patient cannot be used adequately or his physical limitations protected.

The cognitive ability of a stroke patient is a prime consideration. One must know how well he understands oral or written communications. Does he comprehend only short, concrete directions or can he carry through several sequential directions? Are his remarks appropriate or is he operating in an isolated world because of generalized organic brain damage? Is he teachable or incapable of learning?

The side of the brain affected by a stroke is extremely important in assessing cognitive ability because of the special controls in the cerebral hemisphere. The left hemisphere, with its centers for speech and language, controls oral and written communication. The right hemisphere, with its perceptual centers for balance and proprioception, determines how safely and easily the person will handle himself. The right hemisphere also controls perceptual relations of environment and persons, and makes communication through gesture possible when verbal comprehension is in doubt[1].

Knowledge of the person's former life style is crucial to the success of any plan. What was his work history? What were his hobbies, his pleasures? What was his position and role in the family constellation? One's personality usually does not improve after catastrophic illness. In fact, with decreased physical abilities, certain compensatory abilities are lost and some disagreeable traits often become exaggerated. It is extremely difficult to obtain information about life-style and personality from the person and his family, since everyone tends to present the person in the best possible light when there is anxiety in the situation. However, clues to the real person come through regularly and one eventually gains a feeling for him.

After information has been gathered about a patient, problems identified, and judgments made, planning can begin. Judgments about predictable outcomes help in formulating plans. At times, however, information is not precise enough to predict outcomes. The initial plan may be too demanding or not demanding enough. Therefore, a regular evaluation of progress is necessary to keep plans current and appropriate. Keeping plans current may be difficult if many professionals are involved in the therapeutic regimen, especially when a unified approach is required, but all disciplines must communicate freely for the patient's sake.

The teaching plan must be consistent to prevent confusing the patient as well as those working with him. A written teaching plan promotes intelligent implementation.

The following case studies describe adaptations in care for two patients with hemiplegia.

Mr. J. is 58 years old. He sustained a stroke from a right middle cerebral artery thrombosis six weeks ago while working in his machine shop. His general physical condition stabilized quickly, but it took three weeks to reduce his blood pressure to a safe level. He was in an acute-care hospital for five weeks and then moved to an extended care facility.

According to the current assessment of the nursing staff, physical therapist, and physician, Mr. J. has very little physical ability at present. He has been getting out of bed into a chair with the assistance of two and sometimes three people. He weighs 230 lbs., and is six feet, two inches tall. He does not bathe himself, but he does feed himself—and complains about the small portions of his reducing diet. Fortunately he has had no respiratory, skin, bowel, or bladder problems. He has no function in his left arm, but can slide his left leg two to three inches on the bed. He has isolated areas of sensory loss to pain, heat, and cold on his left arm and leg. He knows where they are primarily by looking for them around his left visual field cut.

A driving, gregarious man all his life, Mr. J. ran his machine shop almost single-handedly ten hours a day, six days a week; he bowled twice a week; made repairs on his home; supported three children through their college education; and expected his wife to be a homemaker only. Mr. J. has a quick wit and is pleasant to be with. He believed he could go back to his shop in a couple of weeks after his stroke because he was a strong man who never let an illness keep him down. However, doubts are growing as he lies quietly in bed and gazes into space. He asks each person he sees when his arm and leg will start to move. He learned that the machine shop business has dropped off to practically nothing since neither of his two assistants seems able to make decisions, and he wonders if the business will survive if he does not return soon. He also worries about how his wife will manage if he is no longer the bread winner.

Ms. P., 39 years old, sustained a right-sided hemiplegia from an embolus lodged in her left middle cerebral artery after open-heart surgery for mitral stenosis. The stroke occurred two weeks after surgery when she was preparing to leave the hospital the next day. She was on bedrest one week and spent another week in bed or chair during her anticoagulant therapy. Her medical condition is considered stable with good cardiac function. She has been moved to a rehabilitation unit because of her relatively young age and some spontaneous return of function.

Ms. P.'s assessment by the physician, nurse, and physical therapist shows questionable abilities to date. She has been lifted to the chair by two people. She feeds herself when the food is prepared and placed within her left visual field. She has bathed only her face and chest, has movement in her right shoulder, and can lift her right leg six inches off the bed. She is five feet, two inches tall and weighs 120 lbs. She makes no effort to make a sound, but seems to understand some speech. She has had no swallowing, respiratory, or bowel problems since her stroke, but does have a bladder infection, perhaps from the retention catheter inserted at the time of surgery.

Ms. P. has two sons, 20 and 12, and a 16-year-old daughter. Until last year, when her cardiac problem limited her activities, she cared for her six-room house and helped her husband with the bookkeeping of the shoe store he manages. She was active in the Parent-Teacher Association and church. The family took on the heavier household chores during the past year, but depended on Ms. P.'s decisions.

What professional assessments and judgments can be made about Mr. J. and Ms. P.? Physically, Mr. J's. right side is not disabled and he should eventually have good motion and strength. He has normal cardiac and respiratory function. His intelligence and his sense of humor are intact. His wife needs him and wants him home, and he is strongly motivated to return to work. Work may not be a realistic goal, but, if he masters self-care activities, the team will predict whether work is feasible.

Ms. P. has good left-side function, some right-leg function, and shoulder strength. Her proprioception is probably intact. She was a self-directed person, and her family needs and wants her. Her comprehension and communication are yet to be explored, but indications are that these abilities can be recovered.

Both Mr. J. and Ms. O. have some limited abilities. Other potentials are yet to be discovered. One must never underestimate a person's inner strengths and motivation. To make the most of the new abilities, professionals must use various measures to promote success and limit failures.

IMPLEMENTING CARE

A structured plan based on the application of professional knowledge to a specific problem helps a patient develop skills. It is more satisfying to him if he has identifiable and achievable goals rather than a casual and loosely organized plan. For Mr. J., who has right brain damage, balance and perceptual problems are major limitations to walking, as well as all self care activities. Therefore every means of improving balance and learning perceptual tricks must be employed. Ms. P., on the contrary, has no perceptual problems other than a visual field cut and she should relearn self care and ambulation activities with relative ease.

The learning setting should be quiet, free from distraction, and furnished with equipment suited to the patient. First, Mr. J. and Ms. P. will learn many activities using a bed and chair. The bed should be at a height that permits the person's feet to be placed firmly on the floor when he sits on the side of the bed. The bed must be stable and not move. This may mean taking off wheels or casters. A gatch bed is not necessary. The entire spring and mattress must be firm. A soft mattress decreases balance and an alternating pressure mattress throws a person completely off balance. The bed should be placed so that the patient moves in and out of it from his unaffected side. A trapeze is a hindrance because it keeps a person hanging in mid-air by his unaffected arm and, therefore, he cannot use that side to aid in transfer.

The chair seat should be firm and at the same height as the bed, with arms that extend to the edge of the seat. If a wheelchair is used, it must have brakes that lock. A wheelchair allows the patient to use his available strength most effectively for early mobility. The chair should be placed next to the head of the bed on the patient's noninvolved side. With such an arrangement, Mr. J. can protect his left side better which has areas of sensory loss. Chair placement is important for both Mr. J. and Ms. P., who have reduced visual fields, since it allows them to see what they are doing within the working space. Mr. J.'s field cut is a left hemonymous hemianopsia which gives him half vision of each eye to his right side only. Ms. P.'s visual field problem involves nearly complete loss of vision in her right eye, but complete vision in her left eye.

When the person is ready to dress, he needs large, loose, soft garments with front openings, and well-fitting, sturdy shoes. Wearing loose shoes or slippers or socks only contributes to falls because they do not provide a firm base for standing.

Ms. P. is easily distracted by sounds she does not comprehend. A single room or a two-bed area with a quiet roommate is ideal for her. When faced with a difficult task and questionable success, even someone without brain or other physical impairment is easily distracted. The patient who has a questionable chance for success usually loses interest quickly and shows early signs of fatigue(2). Mr. J.'s and Ms. P.'s attention spans, ability to tolerate failure, and fatigability are unknown, so these aspects must be observed closely, evaluated, and kept to a minimum. When the task is hard, even the smallest failure may cause a person to give up, even if he had been succeeding regularly. Family members or other persons may distract the patient with conversation or ideas contrary to that being taught. Quiet supportive help is needed; distracting people should be asked to leave during a work session.

Teaching should be done at a regular time and preferably by the same person. A hit-or-miss time and person arrangement devalues what is being taught and interferes with continuity and consistency.

The teacher should be alert for fatigue, which may lead to failure. Fatigue may vary from day to day for physical or psychological reasons. The person may slow down, appear distracted, or start to fumble. However, five minutes of good work achieves more than 30 minutes of poor work. The teacher, too, needs a measure of success to encourage the person to try when the task takes extra effort. One should not be overanxious when success comes slowly, especially when the person is starting his program.

Fatigue is not the only reason a patient does not perform. He may be so physically decompensated that he cannot work, even if he strongly desires to. Each day of immobility requires three days of activity to regain the strength and endurance lost(3). A person faints when he attempts to stand after four weeks of recumbency(4). In addition, if contractures develop, it often takes as long as a year to stretch them. For example, when a shoulder is not used but is not immobilized it takes 21 days' exercise to regain full range of shoulder motion; 7 days' immobilization requires 52 days to cover full range of motion; 14 days requires 120 days; and 21 requires 300 or more days(5). Reconditioning calls for increased endurance to overcome fatigue. Muscles tire in direct proportion to their size and use; the larger the muscle, the faster it loses tone. According to Erich Müller, strength is lost at a rate of five percent a day(6).

Strength, endurance, and control are developed by short, sustained, resistive exercises because all muscle fibers have a certain recovery period after contracting before they can contract again(7). The number of fibers contracting depends on the amount of resistance to be overcome. Power develops if the fibers are not excessively stressed and if adequate recovery time is allowed. Therefore any reconditioning program must be started slowly and increased gradually. It is well to perform an active resistive exercise only three or four times at the start of a program. Passive exercise maintains joint mobility only, it does not build strength or endurance. Too vigorous exercise early in the program may cause such great fatigue that the muscles do not recover for several days and the patient's entire program is set back. Muscle fatigue or stress is better controlled with slow sustained exercise so that fatigue can be more easily judged and prevented. Because rapid movements put limited stress on muscles they do not build endurance and are of little value in reconditioning. Mr. J. may be over-eager to exercise because of his desire to return to work, so he will need watching.

Besides deconditioned muscles, the stroke patient has poorly functioning limbs which become extra burdens, literally weights to carry. A person needs adequate strength to handle his body weight. This strength can be the ability to push or to pull a weight in a mechanical fashion to achieve movement. His strength must be at least equal to his total body weight and can be estimated by his ability to push or pull the person testing or by spring-type resistance gauges. Ease of movement grossly indicates a person's strength. The ability to sustain an activity relates to endurance. Mr. J. has 230 pounds to move and he moves in an uncertain manner due to his balance and other perceptual space problems. Ms. P. has only 120 pounds to manage, and she has normal balance and space relations.

Cardiac output in a normal heart lessens with periods of immobility. Normally, the heart responds to the increased demand of tissues for blood with greater stroke volume and moderately increased pulse rate. This response is augmented by the muscle tone in the heart, blood vessels, and skeletal muscles. With decreased tone, these muscles lose their extra propulsion force and, as a result, the pulse rate increases but the delivery of blood to the tissues is limited(8). The person fatigues more quickly as his pulse races. If he has any coronary vessel limitation, he may suffer a heart attack. Mr. J. may be a candidate for a heart attack because he has atherosclerotic disease and has been immobile for six weeks. Ms. P. has had good cardiac function since her surgery, but how great a demand can be placed on it? Demands must be increased slowly and signs of overexertion heeded.

Physical and emotional problems always can arise in any plan for re-education toward independence. Therefore, the plan must be implemented slowly and cautiously at first. The sequence of tasks taught and abilities developed will depend on the total assessment and desires of the patient and his family. Usually, a logical progression can be maintained if the patient and his family are kept informed and involved and if professionals are flexible.

I have found programmed instruction especially valuable in situations where learning takes place over a long period. I developed programmed instruction material for stroke patients to teach bed mobility, transfers, and dressing with one hand, and tested its use in a limited study. The practicality of teaching by this method was measured by the number of trials required to learn an activity. Patients in the experimental group receiving progressive, step-by-step instruction averaged one trial per task, while patients in the control group required one-and-a-half to ten trials, the average patient requiring three. Observations of the control group indicated that failure was due to lack of readiness to perform a task. In addition, different tasks were taught by different people at various times with little or no communication between the teachers. The test group, which learned with the help of one person at specific times, required 6 to 26 sessions of programmed instruction to learn tasks. The control subjects required from 15 to 40. The test group sessions ranged from 15 to 75 minutes while the control group sessions lasted from 10 to 45 minutes.

Patients like Mr. J. with dubious prospects for success need a well-planned and executed program. The Ms. P.s can also benefit from a well-structured plan which enables them to learn an activity with less trial and error.

The often overwhelming depression and concrete thinking that accompany strokes cannot be ignored when one is helping a patient develop a new self-image. One's directions must be concrete and precise, without metaphors, allusions, or comparisons. Slower comprehension often accompanies concrete thinking, so all communication should be in short sentences that present only one idea at a time(9). However, the language must be appropriate for adults. Speaking to Mr. J., for instance, in terms suitable for a child would be very degrading and might increase his depression.

Depression is common among stroke patients and others with chronic irreversible problems. However, depression can be a favorable prognostic sign as it indicates that the person is facing reality, an absolute necessity if he is to take part in a program. Helping him succeed in tasks which make for independence helps alleviate his depression so that he can discover new values and self-worth. Usually, the longer a person remains dependent the more depressed he becomes and the more difficult it is to relieve depression(10). However, the moment of readiness to participate varies markedly—a fact that professionals should consider in all planning and care. A stroke patient needs active treatment as soon as possible to lessen not only the effects of physical immobility but also the effects of depression.

EVALUATION

Every care plan must provide regular times for evaluation to determine if particular techniques are effective or if other methods should be introduced. Usually changes are made when a plan does not work. It is equally important to recognize an effective method so that appropriate parts can be used in other areas with the patient. Regular, systematic evaluation times will establish the rate of change and progress for the patient and the professionals. Evaluation entails reassessment of strengths and weaknesses as well as identification of other problems that arise. These determinations help the patient and the team to adjust and set goals appropriate to his progress.

The nursing process applies not only to the beginning stages of living with a disability but to the many years that follow. In the second and third years after a stroke, the person feels the full impact of his disability. Friends who once helped withdraw and family members must find other means of assistance or become so fatigued they need a respite from their burdens.

With the support of local heart associations, several communities have organized community stroke groups for socialization. These enable individuals to find out more about living with their strokes, and provide opportunities to put a little fun into their lives with picnics, outings to the theatre, the horse races, and so on. After these experiences, many patients and their relatives have been willing to return to former activities.

Professional attention by all disciplines, nursing in particular, can direct a scientifically based plan of care for and with the stroke patient. Careful assessment, identification of problems with planning of sequential goals, implementation suited to the patient, and regular evaluation offer victims the opportunity to live to their fullest.

REFERENCES

1. FOWLER, R. S., AND FORDYCE, W. E. Adapting care for the brain-damaged patient. *Am.J.Nurs.* 72:1832-1835, Oct. 1972.
2. BENTON, A. L. Motivational influences on performance of brain-damaged patients. Brain and behavior symposium II. *Am.J. Ortho-psychiatry* 30:315-321, Apr. 1960.
3. KOTTKE, F. J. The effects of limitation of activity upon the human body. *JAMA* 196: 826, June 6, 1966.
4. MOIDEL, H. C., AND OTHERS, EDS. *Nursing Care of the Patient*

with *Medical-Surgical Disorders*. New York, McGraw-Hill Book Co., 1971, p. 409.
5. KRUSEN, F. H., AND OTHERS, EDS. *Handbook of Physical Medicine and Rehabilitation*. Philadelphia, Pa., W. B. Saunders Co., 1965, pp. 368-369.
6. MULLER, E. A. Influence of training and of inactivity on muscle strength. *Arch.Phys.Med.Rehabil.* 51:449, Aug. 1970.
7. GUYTON, A. C. *Textbook of Medical Physiology*. 3d ed. Philadelphia, W. B. Saunders Co., 1966, p. 99.
8. *Ibid.*, p. 339.
9. FOWLER AND FORDYCE, *op.cit*, p. 1833.
10. REITAN, R. M. Qualitative versus quantitative mental changes following brain damage. *J. Psychol.* 46:339-346, 1958.

Soft or Hard Devices to Position Hands?

NANCY DAYHOFF

A familiar nursing practice is reexamined on the basis of pathophysiology.

Too often, nursing procedures are based on intuitive thinking or environmental work pressures rather than established knowledge(1). Constant use of a nursing technique may breed a false sense of security about its therapeutic value, a sense not justified by theoretical rationale or clinical exploration of the technique. This is evident in the lack of literature dealing with research on the common nursing interventions to prevent the "hemiplegia fist" or "claw-hand deformity" in adults who have had diseases resulting in brain damage.

Nurses who care for hemiplegic patients know the importance of positioning to prevent deformity. Almost every nursing book or article stresses the use of mechanical devices during the acute and rehabilitative phases of care, usually ones that are soft and bulky, such as rolled washcloths, gauze, or sponge rubber(2-13). Assuming that some positioning device will be beneficial for a patient, I suggest that a device that is different from those generally used may be more effective in preventing deformity.

One of the earliest articles in the nursing literature, in 1941, showed nine illustrations of the proper positioning of patients. Four pictures showed a hand positioned with a rolled bandage. In discussing the importance of positioning to prevent contractures, the author stated that muscle contractures with deformity occur as a result of prolonged positioning that favors one muscle group(2). No reference was made to the

---

MS. DAYHOFF, *R.N., M.S., M.Ed.*, is an associate professor of nursing, Indiana University School of Nursing, Indiana University—Purdue University at Indianapolis.

contribution of spasticity to deformities or to the direct effects of the bandage in the prevention of contractures. Current pictures resemble those in that 1941 article.

Discussions have continued to center on the idea that fibers of overactive muscles become permanently shortened, that these muscles then exert a greater pull on the joints than the weaker muscles, and that the weaker muscles become permanently lengthened. Since the flexor muscles of the hands are more powerful than the extensor muscles, the typical picture of the paralyzed hand is one of extreme flexion or the claw-hand deformity(6). How a soft hand-positioning device either interrupts the overactivity or prevents the shortening of muscles is not discussed. Without regard for the underlying pathophysiology, authors assume that soft devices maintain a desirable anatomical position.

It is possible, I believe, that a soft hand-positioning device may contribute to flexion of the hand. Soft objects placed in an infant's hand stimulate the palmar-grasp reflex. This reflex becomes inhibited as the infant matures(14-16). However, in brain-damaged persons, this primitive reflex may reappear and soft hand rolls may encourage palmar-grasp reaction(17).

All hemiplegic patients tend to follow specific stages of recovery. Immediately after the cerebral insult, the hemiplegia may be flaccid(18). Few patients remain at this level. In the arm, wrist, and fingers, mass reactions and reflex activity often occur and become manifest as flexion synergy. Any willed movement of the upper extremity results in some degree of flexion, adduction, and internal rotation of the shoulder, wrist, and fingers. The joint movements become limited(16,19,20).

If a device could inhibit the hypertonia of the wrist and finger flexors, perhaps the extensor muscles would become more effective. This might decrease flexor hyperactivity and produce a more functional hand. Ayres, Farber, and Stockmeyer suggest using a hard palmar hand-positioning device to inhibit the hypertonia of the fingers (21-23). They recommend that the device provide constant pressure over the entire flexor (palmar) surface of the fingers and be firm enough to provide total contact over the palmar surface without stretching the spastic fingers. The theoretical rationale for such a device is under investigation.

I worked with three patients in a convalescent center to examine the clinical effectiveness of a hard hand-positioning device. These patients had had cerebral vascular insults several years previously. At the time of the study, no hand-positioning devices were being used, no exercises were being done, and flexion deformities were evident.

The hand-positioning device I used with them was a cone made of

CONTEMPORARY NURSING SERIES

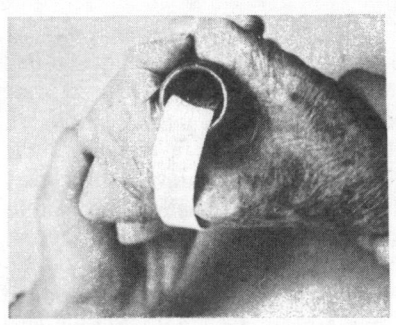

A hard hand-positioning device such as this might decrease flexor activity and increase hand function.

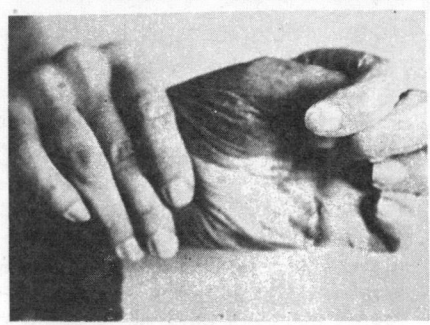

Flexion contractures of the fingers as shown here are typical of the deformity hemiplegic patients experience.

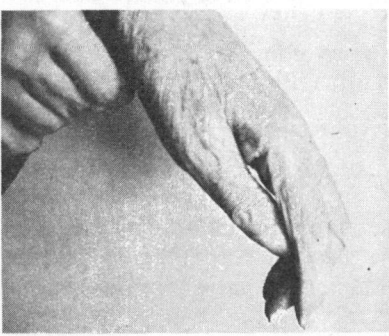

Improvement in the patient's ability to extend his fingers can be seen in photo taken after 20 weeks' use of hard hand-positioning device.

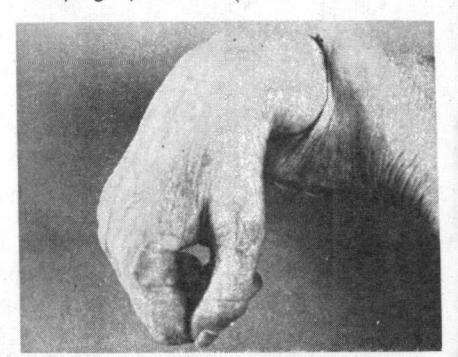

Some passive finger extension could be achieved with the wrist flexed after this patient used a hard hand-positioning device for four weeks.

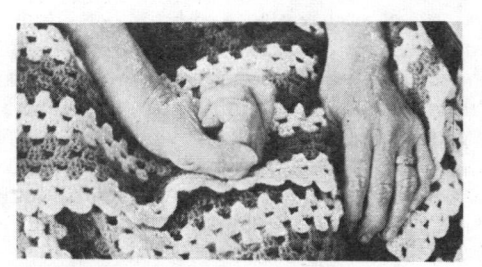

Both wrist- and finger-flexion contractures occur when a patient's hand remains positioned as below.

227

firm cardboard with a circumference of approximately six and one-half inches at the large end and four inches at the narrow end. This size cone exerts constant pressure over the flexor surface of the palm and fingers. A broad elastic band over the dorsal surface of the fingers holds the device in place. The elastic band is tight enough to maintain the cone's contact on the flexor surface but not tight enough to cause pressure areas on the skin. The patients used those cones throughout the day except during hygienic procedures and removed them at night.

I made weekly assessments of hand position and function, using a Hines Digit-O-Meter and a Jamar Dynamometer. Originally the patients were to be followed for six weeks, but because of the positive results during this period, I continued periodic measurements for one year.

The Digit-O-Meter was used to assess the amount of passive extension of the fingers(24). The meter was placed on the palmar crease and the fingers were passively extended to the point of maximum resistance. This yielded data concerning composite extension. Finger extension in relation to thumb opposition was tested by placing the meter along the medial aspect of the thumb and the tip of each finger individually. These two aspects of extension were measured first with the wrist flexed and then with the wrist in neutral position.

The Dynamometer was used to measure grip force in pounds(25). With his arm in any position he chose that was not in contact with his body, the patient was given two opportunities to exert his most forceful grip. The maximum grip force was recorded.

Mr. A., 84-years old, had a left hemiplegia and was confined to a wheelchair when out of bed. He reported that his hand had become increasingly useless following his stroke seven years before. His fingers were contracted into the palm of his hand. His elbow was usually held in a flexed position although he could extend it slightly. After baseline data were obtained, the cone was placed in his affected hand.

At the end of six weeks, Mr. A. had full passive extension of his little finger with his wrist flexed; and the passive extension of his first three fingers had improved considerably. However, with his wrist in neutral position, his fingers showed less improvement. He could not extend his fingers and, according to the Dynamometer measurements, he had made little progress in gaining a functional grip. The maximum range of active finger extension he achieved (with wrist flexed) after 20 weeks can be seen on page 227 (middle photograph).

Slight active extension of his wrist was evident by the sixth week and still present one year later. His grasp ability showed little improvement at the end of a year when compared to measurement after the sixth week.

The difference between the finger extension achieved with the wrist flexed and with the wrist in neutral position is an example of the synergistic movement resulting from brain damage.

Ms. B., 75-years old, had a right hemiplegia and some motor aphasia which resulted from her CVA of five years before. She was confined to a wheelchair because of a below-the-knee amputation. She constantly held her hand in her lap with her forearm supinated; her wrist and fingers were acutely flexed. Ms. B. continued to hold her hand in supination even after the cone was used and refused to place her hand prone even for short periods.

With her wrist flexed, Ms. B. showed improvement in passive finger extension. When Ms. B.'s wrist was placed in neutral position, however, her flexed fingers resisted passive manipulation. She showed no evidence of active extension of her wrist or fingers and no grasp ability. One year later, after continuous use of the cone, some deterioration was seen.

Ms. C., who was 84-years old, had had multiple strokes over several years. She was semiconscious. While there was no indication in her medical record that she was hemiplegic, her right hand on baseline evaluation was more resistant to manipulation than her left. I placed a hard cone in her right hand and used nothing in her left hand. Following the second week of my study, the nursing home staff put rolled washcloths in her left hand.

Ms. C.'s right hand showed a small improvement with the hard hand cone. Her less affected, or left, hand showed slight deterioration after the washcloths were begun, especially in the measurements of opposition.

Positive clinical effects could be seen in all three patients after the hard hand-positioning device had been used, even though their fists had been hemiplegic for several years. Maximum improvement was reached by the sixth week. These patients were not in any exercise program.

Although my investigation included only three patients and many variables were not controlled, I believe that serious questions should be directed toward the common nursing practice of using soft hand-positioning devices. A more critical evaluation of the effectiveness of both soft and hard positioning devices might answer such questions as these: Do hand-positioning devices have a desirable effect on the patient? What kind of hand-positioning device yields the most desirable results? Are there any other nursing techniques that affect the outcomes with positioning devices?

Little attention is given to traditional nursing procedures. But these practices may need to be revised in light of new scientific discoveries and closer examination of the clinical effectiveness of practice.

REFERENCES

1. LINDEMAN, C. A., AND VAN AERNAM, BETTY. Nursing intervention with presurgical patients—effects of structured and unstructured preoperative teaching. *Nurs.Res.* 20:319-332. July-Aug. 1971.
2. ALLEN, KATHERINE. Posture and the bed patient. *Am.J.Nurs.* 41:1137-1140, Oct. 1941.
3. FUNSTEN, R. V., AND CALDERWOOD, CARMELITA. *Orthopedic Nursing.* 2nd ed. St. Louis. C. V. Mosby Co., 1949.
4. LARSON, C. B., AND GOULD, MARJORIE. *Calderwood's Orthopedic Nursing.* 5th ed. St. Louis. C. V. Mosby Co., 1961.
5. TERRY, F. J., AND OTHERS. *Principles and Technics of Rehabilitation Nursing.* 2d ed. St. Louis, C. V. Mosby Co., 1961.
6. MORRISSEY, A. B. *Rehabilitation Nursing.* New York, G. P. Putnam's Sons. 1951.
7. PIERSOL, G. M. The nurse in physical medicine. *Am.J.Nurs.* 45:526-531. July 1945.
8. RECOB, M. T. Physical therapy for the stroke patient. *Nurs. Homes* 15:21-25, July 1966.
9. RUSK, H. A. *Rehabilitation Medicine.* 3d ed. St. Louis, C. V. Mosby Co., 1971.
10. SMITH, D. W., AND GERMAIN, C. P. H. *Nursing of Adults.* Philadelphia. J. B. Lippincott Co., 1972.
11. SMITH, D. W., AND OTHERS. *Care of the Adult Patient.* 3d ed. Philadelphia. J. B. Lippincott Co., 1971.
12. SMITH, G. W. *Care of the Patient with a Stroke.* rev. ed. New York. Springer Publishing Co., 1967.
13. THORPE, E. L. M., AND COULL, E. G. Nursing the patient with cerebrovascular accident. *Can.Nurse* 62:38-41. May 1966.
14. MCGRAW, M. B. *The Neuromuscular Maturation of the Human Infant.* New York. Hafner Pub. Co., 1963. (Reprint of 1945 edition)
15. TWITCHELL, T. E. Normal motor development. IN *The Child with Central Nervous System Deficit, Report of Two Symposiums, 1965.* (U.S. Children's Bureau Publication No. 432) Washington, D.C., U.S. Government Printing Office, 1966, pp. 85-89.
16. MAGEE, K. R. Clinical analysis of reflexes. IN *Handbook of Clinical Neurology,* ed. by P. J. Vinken and G. W. Bruyn, New York, American Elsevier Publishing Co., 1969, Vol. 1.
17. SHAHANI, BHAGWAN, AND OTHERS. The grasp reflex and preservation. *Brain* 93:181-192, 1970.
18. PERRY, C. E. Principles and techniques of the Brunnstrom approach to the treatment of hemiplegia. *Am.J.Phys.Med.* 46:789-812. Feb. 1967.
19. NEWMAN, MICHAEL. The process of recovery after hemiplegia. *Stroke* 3:702-710. Nov.-Dec. 1972.
20. TWITCHELL, T. E. The restoration of motor function following hemiplegia in man. *Brain* 74:443-480. Dec. 1951.
21. AYRES, A. J. Integration of information. IN *Approaches to the Treatment of Patients with Neuromuscular Dysfunction.* Proceedings of the Third International Congress of the World Federation of Occupational Therapists, held in Philadelphia. 1962. William C. Brown Co., Dubuque, Iowa.

22. Farber, S. D. *Sensorimotor Evaluation and Treatment Procedures for Allied Health Personnel.* Indiana University-Purdue University at Indianapolis, Medical Center, Indiana Univ. Foundation. Indianapolis, 1973.
23. Stockmeyer, S. A. An interpretation of the approach of Rood to the treatment of neuromuscular dysfunction. *Am.J.Phys.Med.* 49:900-961. Feb. 1967.
24. Brayman, Sara. Measuring device for joint motion of the hand. *Am.J.Occup.Ther.* 25:173. Apr. 1971.
25. Sister Kenny Institute. *Technical Manual-Hand Strength and Dexterity Tests,* by Marjorie Kellor and others. Minneapolis. The Institute 1971.

Feeding Techniques for Dysphagic Patients

TERRY WEILER GAFFNEY
ROSEMARY PETERSON CAMPBELL

Brain-injured patients must relearn lip closure, sucking, and swallowing before they can eat successfully. Stimulation techniques aid in this process.

Stimulating a patient who has central nervous system damage to eat as normally as possible is a challenging nursing problem. When a patient who has been receiving tube feedings begins oral intake, attempts to feed him frequently are met with frustration and failure.

Nurses can stimulate normal eating patterns by applying the same techniques occupational therapists use in working with brain-damaged children. In many instances, such stimulation may replace the need for nasogastric and gastrostomy feeding tubes. This approach to feeding is based on stimulating those receptors which enhance lip closure, sucking, and swallowing.

Before introducing food, identify the special problems which interfere with the person's normal intake. If he has neurological damage which affects his ability to eat and drink, determine what he is able to do and what he cannot do.

Does he have head control? Because eating requires great concentra-

---

MS. GAFFNEY (St. Elizabeth School of Nursing, Lincoln, Neb.; B.S.N., St. Louis University, St. Louis, Mo.; M.S.N., Marquette University, Milwaukee, Wis.) is an instructor, Department of Comparative Nursing Care Systems, University of Washington School of Nursing, Seattle. MS. CAMPBELL (B.S., St. Mary's College, Notre Dame, Ind.; M.S.N., New York Medical College, Graduate School of Nursing, New York) is an instructor in human services at Golden West College, Huntington Beach, Calif.

tion and effort, one should not insist on voluntary head control at mealtime. If the patient has not developed head control and his head falls toward the chest, his head can be stabilized by applying a hand to his forehead. The head should face forward rather than to the side and should not be thrown backward. Some patients tend to throw their heads back to aid in the propulsion of food. Aspiration is likely to occur when the neck is extended in this fashion.

Which position facilitates eating? Positioning the patient in a semireclining position, either in bed or in a wheelchair, will support his head and counteract hyperextension. Some therapists recommend this position because feeding is a flexion-patterned activity. In this posture, less resistance is exerted on the muscles used for eating. Tilting the head forward slightly reduces the possibility of aspiration(1).

Can he open his mouth? Occasionally a patient cannot open his mouth voluntarily. Attempting to force his jaw open only strengthens closure. The triggering device for mouth opening is at the lips. To get the patient started, lightly touch both his lips with the tip of a spoon(2). If his mouth does not open after this stimulus, use a finger to apply light pressure on the chin just below the lower lip. Ask the patient to open at the same time. Stroking the digastric muscle—the V-shaped muscle under the chin—without crossing the midline also stimulates opening.

Can he bring his lips together and close his mouth? Successful feeding techniques depend on lip closure. Most people cannot swallow without first closing their lips. If a person cannot approximate his lips, several techniques can be tried to stimulate closure. Stroke the lips with a finger or an ice popsicle three or four times. Or apply manual pressure just above the upper lip, using the thumb and forefinger or the side of a finger.

Can he purse his lips as in a sucking gesture? A person who cannot use his lips to remove food from a spoon needs help to strengthen sucking. To stimulate more effective closure, a small disc fitted around a short straw provides sensory stimulation when placed at the lips. Longer straws and thicker liquids can be used progressively. Sucking depends on lip closure and tongue position.

Can he move his tongue in all planes? Normally, the tongue is positioned at the floor of the mouth during sucking. If there is limited tongue

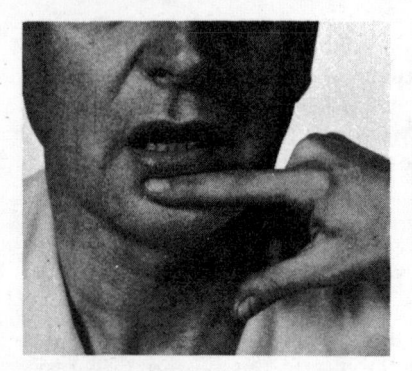

To stimulate mouth opening apply light pressure on the chin.

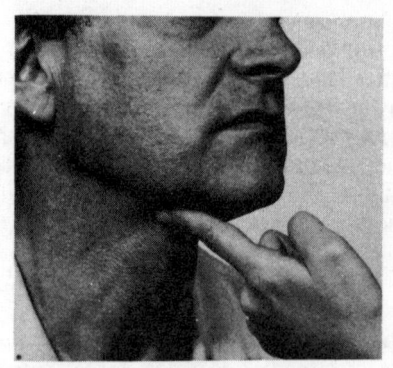

Or, stroke the digastric muscle beneath the chin.

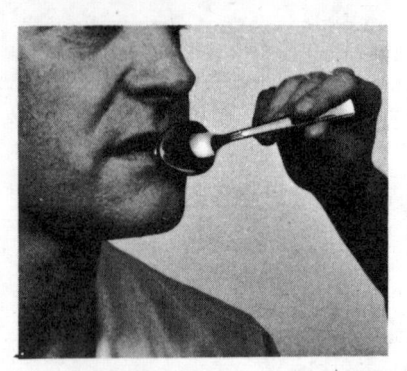

Touching lips with spoon also may stimulate opening.

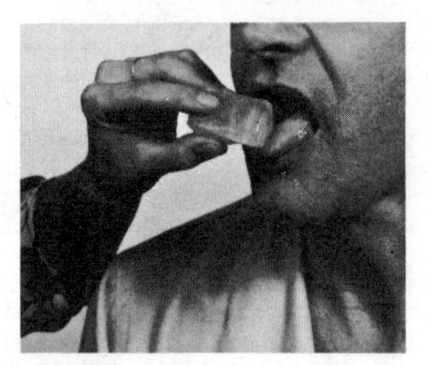

Ice tongue to enhance its mobility.

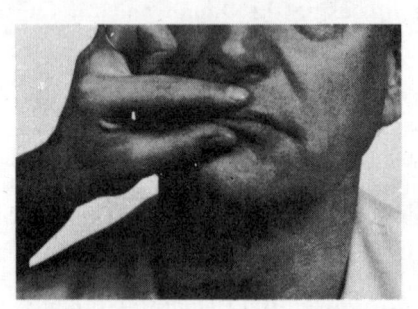

Pressure above lip stimulates closure.

movement, touch a tongue blade lightly to the tissue just behind the lower teeth. This stimulation, which can be applied to any part of the mouth where you want the tongue to move, facilitates tongue movement in any plane. Icing weak tongue muscles also enhances tongue mobility.

If tongue protrusion interferes with eating, apply pressure on the soft tissue under the mandible. Walking a tongue blade from the tip to the back of the tongue will inhibit tongue thrust and stifle the gag reflex.

Is saliva being secreted? When salivary flow is decreased, icing with a flavored popsicle stimulates the salivary glands. If the person drools, plain ice is preferred.

Can he swallow? An environment relatively free of distracting stimuli is especially important for persons with dysphagia. Concentration and effort are required to promote swallowing and overcome the fears associated with dysphagia. Icing the sternal notch and briskly rubbing the back of the neck near the occiput with a terrycloth washcloth will stimulate swallowing.

Food must look, smell, and taste good. The person should be given the opportunity to see and smell his food. Bring the spoon into his visual field and ask him to savor the aroma. This will stimulate salivary flow and prepare him for swallowing. Food which is prepared attractively looks more palatable. Pureed foods do not provide the sensory satisfactions that fork-mashed vegetables, fruits, and finely cut meats do. Cold or hot liquids stimulate sensory receptors more than tepid fluids do.

If the person is to eat successfully at home, his family members must observe and participate in feeding techniques. Sometimes only two or three stimulation methods will be enough to accomplish the desired results. By assisting with feeding before discharge, the family member learns which techniques work most effectively with his relative. As a further support, the steps they should follow can be listed and illustrated with pictures.

These techniques were modified and applied successfully in the care of an elderly woman. Ms. P. had suffered several respiratory arrests and had resultant paralysis of muscles of the lips, tongue, palate, and larynx. Her abilities were assessed, and then a management program was planned which included clamping her gastrostomy tube and giving her supplementary intravenous fluids.

After icing her lips, the nurse spooned ice chips into her mouth to provide general sensory stimulation five times daily. Ms. P. was told to hold the ice in her mouth for a few seconds and then expel it. She would then take a teaspoon of ice chips, chew for a few seconds, identify the sensations of cold and wet, think swallow, and finally swallow slowly and deliberately. Occasionally, a slight pinch to the larynx facilitated swallowing.

After two days on this regimen, Ms. P. progressed to frozen orange-juice chips and finely cut canned fruits, following the same sequence as in the initial ice regime. As her confidence and success increased with each of the foods, she was given a mechanical diet. After one and a half weeks, she requested fresh cantaloupe, which she ate with little difficulty. Ms. P. then returned home for a weekend visit and ate whatever she liked. The following Monday she was delighted to tell us that even popcorn had posed no problem for her.

Careful assessment of lip closure, sucking, and swallowing and application of techniques developed by other disciplines provide alternatives to trial and error methods of promoting patient feeding. While success cannot be expected in all instances, these feeding approaches may provide more satisfaction for patients.

REFERENCES

1. LARSEN, G. L. Rehabilitation for dysphagia paralytica. *J.Speech Hear.Disord.* 37:187-194. May 1972.
2. HOLSER-BEUHLER, PATRICIA. The Blanchard method of feeding the cerebral palsied. *Am. J.Occup.Ther.* 20:31-34, Jan.-Feb. 1966.

Working with Dysphasic Patients

LINDA HAGEN BELT

Because she has such close contact with patients, the nurse's role in language retraining is a vital one.

When my nursing instructor assigned me to care for a patient with expressive dysphasia, I was elated! Here was an opportunity to use some of the techniques I had learned as a speech therapy student. The patient was an elderly man whose communication disorder was the result of a cerebrovascular accident. Using my speech science background as a starting point, I was able to develop approaches to his care which enabled us to engage in several meaningful and beneficial conversations.

Although a formal speech therapy program should not be initiated by the nurse, she can, under the guidance of a qualified speech therapist, cooperate in the patient's speech therapy program to reinforce and enhance language retraining.

Wepman has defined aphasia as

any language problem resulting from organic disturbance of cortical tissue in which the defect is not due to faulty innervation of the musculature of speech, dysfunction of the peripheral sense organs, or general mental deficiency. The language problem manifests itself in the areas of symbolization, comprehension, and reproduction of concepts while the individual is using or attempting to use conventional spoken or written symbols(1).

MS. BELT *is studying for a B.S.N. at the University of Arizona, Tucson. She has a B.A. degree in speech and hearing sciences from the University of Arizona. The author thanks Rose Gerber, instructor in nursing, and Marcia Campbell, instructor in speech pathology, both of the University of Arizona.*

Aphasia is a disorder in a person's ability to understand and effectively use the symbols that comprise language. This disorder may be secondary to a cerebrovascular accident, a traumatic head injury, or other cerebral disorder. Expressive and receptive dysphasias vary in severity. Although dysphasia may be expressive *or* receptive, concurrent involvement is more common even though one deficiency may be very slight(2).

Aphasia is not dysarthria or apraxia, not a hearing disorder, nor regression to a lower level of intelligence. Dysarthria and apraxia often accompany the aphasias, but should not be confused with the specific disorders of symbolic processing.

Aphasia in and of itself usually does not delay a person's recovery from stroke. But without intervention by those who are caring for him, the effects of aphasia on the patient can be devastating(3). He may feel humiliated, totally withdraw, and cease attempts to speak; in extreme cases a person may lose his will to live(4). These are the specific objectives for care of the expressive dysphasic patient:

- an understanding by involved staff of the nature of dysphasia and its effects on the patient
- establishing a means for the patient to communicate his basic needs to staff
- providing an atmosphere conducive to communication
- encouraging the patient in his efforts to communicate.

Basic to all interactions and care provided for the expressive dysphasic patient is the fact that he is an *adult*. When a person develops a communication disorder, it is all too easy for those around him to think of him as having lost part of his intellectual ability or having regressed to an earlier developmental stage. This is not the case. The expressive dysphasic patient's problem lies in the area of symbolic processing. He must be accepted and treated as an adult at all times.

COMMUNICATING BASIC NEEDS

Every person must be able to communicate his basic needs to those around him. For the expressive dysphasic patient, this presents a definite problem. Because he has difficulty with verbal communication, the nurse must assume more responsibility for assessing his needs. She should become familiar with his gestures, especially his eye signals and she must be very consistent in her own communication(5). If necessary, a system of signals should be worked out with the patient. For example, he can shake his head to indicate "no" and nod for "yes."

In assessing basic needs, the nurse should phrase her questions so that they cannot be misunderstood, speak directly to the patient, and enunciate clearly. When she interprets the person's body language, she should consistently validate her interpretation with the person so that she avoids the possibility of misinterpretations.

Conveying basic needs will be easier for the patient if the nurse anticipates them. In this way he is not forced to make repeated attempts at asking for things. Therefore, observation skills are vital. The patient should be checked frequently for signs of pain, for discomfort due to room temperature, wrinkled or soiled linens, or a need to be repositioned, and for evidence of the need to urinate or defecate. Medication orders, especially for analgesics, exercise and skin care regimens, and other regular procedures should be carried out on schedule.

NON-LANGUAGE CHARACTERISTICS

Once the patient and the nurse have established a means of communication, the nurse should work toward creating an atmosphere in which the patient can "relearn" language. Attention must be given to the patient's non-language characteristics. According to Wepman,

the brain defect which produces the aphasia is seen to produce also many other far reaching symptoms beyond the realm of language. Many personality aberrations, many atypical modes of behavior that are not readily acceptable in our society, and various other symptoms of a functional nature are seen to be the direct or indirect result of the cerebral impairment . . . maximal success in therapy can only be obtained when it includes due consideration of the personality of the patient and the appearance of behavioral aberrations.(6).

Six commonly encountered, problem-causing, non-language characteristics that may develop are emotional lability, frustration with cluttered situations, visual defects, fecal incontinence, paresis or paralysis, and forgetfulness.

Emotional lability is frustrating for both patient and nurse, and is manifested most dramatically by the patient's tendency to burst into tears frequently and for no apparent reason. This problem is often associated with dysphasia(3). The nurse must expect inconsistencies in the patient's day-to-day performance. When these sudden changes of behavior do occur, they should be accepted as normal. When crying spells occur, the most appropriate nursing action is to ignore the outburst and let the patient cry it out. Too much sympathy will usually prolong the outburst, and this is not helpful to him(7).

Dysphasic patients often become frustrated in cluttered surroundings. They are also upset by changes in the arrangement of furniture and personal belongings(8). Therefore, the nurse should pay particular attention to keeping the patient's room as tidy as possible, with the furniture in its usual place. A patient who wants his water pitcher and drinking glass arranged in a particular way on the bedside table is usually very willing to show where, even if only by pointing. While this may sound time-consuming and relatively insignificant, it is easily taken care of and definitely helps create an atmosphere conducive to communication.

The remaining non-language characteristics are not behavioral aberrations as such; they have organic bases. Failure to intervene, however, can cause communication problems. Visual disturbance is a common aftermath of head injury, and usually occurs on the contralateral side. The nurse should always approach the patient from his unaffected side and be sure that his bed is positioned so that his unaffected eye faces the entrance to the room. Many patients have exaggerated startle responses when others approach them from their "blind" side. This often upsets them so much that meaningful language interaction can be lost.

Fecal incontinence is embarrassing and frustrating for anyone, but is even more upsetting to the dysphasic patient. Hygienic care after defecation must be carried out promptly with no facial or verbal indication of displeasure. Frustration is the worst enemy of the dysphasic, and any embarrassment can cause him to withdraw and cease communication attempts(8).

Hemiplegia is another common result of cortical damage. This can range from mild paresis to paralysis. To help relieve anxiety about this problems, the nurse should praise and encourage any progress the patient makes in regaining function; the smallest amount of progress is vitally important to him. She should participate actively in his exercise program and should keep in touch with the physician and physical therapist regarding changes in or additions to it. Even shaking hands with the patient rather than just saying hello can be helpful.

Dysphasic patients with bilateral lesions are often forgetful. The patient may indicate that he understands the nurse's instructions, but may fail to carry them out. He understands, he wants to cooperate, but he forgets easily. This behavior is normal; the patient needs to be reminded frequently of things he must do(8).

APPROACHES

To encourage the patient's communication efforts, the nurse should provide meaningful auditory input for him and meaningful responses to his attempts at communication.

Auditory stimulation is a primary need of the person with expressive dysphasia while he is relearning symbolic language(7). Each time the nurse speaks to him, she provides both stimulation and an example. Therefore, she should speak clearly, always look directly at him, enunciate each word, and use a normal level of loudness. The fact that a person cannot answer very well does not mean that he cannot hear(9). Getting "hollered at" is very frustrating. Also, care should be taken to avoid discussing the patient with other persons when he can overhear what is being said about him.

The dysphasic patient requires time to process incoming stimuli. Therefore, one should speak slowly. While giving routine care, an extra five or ten minutes should be taken to avoid conveying the idea that the nurse is rushed; if the patient feels rushed, he may not attempt to communicate. All procedures should be explained thoroughly, but only one idea should be presented at a time.

Social communication can be established by telling the person what is going on in the hospital and the world outside. This relieves his feelings of isolation and encourages social communication attempts(9). If he points to something, such as a glass of water, provide auditory stimulation by saying, "Do you want a glass of water?" He may not respond verbally, but the auditory stimulation is vitally important.

Chattering should be avoided. It is confusing and frustrating because it provides too much stimulation for the person to process at one time. Double-barreled questions should also be avoided. He can be confused about which question to answer first, and the integration and formulation of two different sets of information is a perplexing task. When several questions must be asked, the best approach is to use simple "yes-no" questions. This information is processed more readily and if the patient is able to respond, he experiences the success which is so vital to his continued efforts to speak.

In order to respond meaningfully to the dysphasic patient's communication, the nurse must give him every opportunity to communicate(2). Patience is the key word—patience in allowing the dysphasic person time to speak, and patience in understanding his garbled speech. He needs time to retrieve words and formulate ideas and should never be given the impression that the nurse does not have time to listen. Also, he should be praised and encouraged for each *attempt* at communications as well as for each *success*.

While he should be given every opportunity to speak, the dysphasic patient should never be *expected* to say anything. For these patients, speech inconsistencies are as common as behavioral inconsistencies, and the ability to say a word or phrase one day does not mean that he can do so the next. Comments like "But you said it yesterday" only foster frustration.

If the person appears to be having trouble finding a word, it should not be supplied for him immediately. Often our guesses are not accurate and this upsets the patient. If his repeated attempts are beginning to upset him, he can be offered a multiple choice of words.

Complex or long conversations should be avoided because dysphasic patients tire easily. Frequent, five minute conversations are much more beneficial. Many patients curse suddenly for no apparent reason. This is part of the automatic language function that most dysphasic patients retain, not an attack on the nurse, and should be accepted as such(9). A final point is that any display of amusement at a patient's communication attempts should be avoided. Dysphasic speech is often humorous, but laughter only embarrasses the patient and thwarts further communication attempts.

Consistency in approach and day-by-day stimulation of communication by the nurse augment the formal language retraining the patient receives and can speed the reestablishment of effective communication.

REFERENCES

1. WEPMAN, J. M. *Recovery from Aphasia.* New York, Ronald Press Co., 1951, p. 4.
2. BOONE, D. R. *Adult Has Aphasia.* Danville, Ill., Interstate Printers and Publishers, 1965, pp. 3-24.
3. HELPING the stroke patient to come back. *Nurs.Update* 2:1, 3-7, Apr. 1971.
4. DAVIS, R. W. Communication with the stroke victim. *Bedside Nurse* 3:24-26, Dec. 1970.
5. HALPER, A. S., AND OTHERS. Communication problems of the stroke patient. *Nurs.Homes* 16:17-19, Oct. 1967.
6. WEPMAN, *op.cit.,* p. 4, 19.
7. MILLER, B. E. Assisting aphasic patients with speech rehabilitation. *Am.J.Nurs.* 69:984, May 1969.
8. BUCK, MCKENSIE. *Dysphasia: Professional Guidance for Family and Patient.* Englewood Cliffs, N.J., Prentic-Halle, 1968, pp. 30-34.
9. FOX, M. J. Talking with patients who can't answer. *Am.J.Nurs.* 71:1146-1148, June 1971.

Aphasic Patients Talk Back

MADGE SKELLY

The aphasic patient's inability to respond may be related more to environment than to brain damage.

The adult who is aphasic encounters many frustrating situations in which people treat him as if he were stupid, drunk, childish, imbecilic, psychotic, or a combination of these. Well-meaning attempts are made to impose unprofitable drills on him, frequently patterned on procedures for children or for mentally retarded persons. Some professional people use behavior approaches toward the aphasic adult which cause him to regress, seldom assist him to communicate, and almost always add to his already severe frustration. Often these approaches are used because the results of research on aphasia are unknown.

Findings of a recent project may provide nurses with additional background and information for improving the human environment of aphasic patients. We interviewed 50 aphasic patients who had recovered a useful level of speech. All had been classified as severely impaired on admission. Structured questions and open-end topics were presented. Free flow of opinion and feeling was encouraged. We analyzed all the interview content and identified 12 areas of unanimous, serious concern to aphasic patients.

ABILITY TO COMPREHEND All who were interviewed stated emphatically that they understood what was said in their presence much sooner and

---

MADGE SKELLY, PH.D. *is chief, Audiology and Speech Pathology Service, Veterans Administration Hospital, St. Louis, Mo.; professor of communication disorders, St. Louis University Graduate School; and professor of community medicine, St. Louis Univ. School of Medicine. This research was supported by St. Louis Veterans Administration Hospital Research Funds, MRIS 8100.*

much more completely than the literature on aphasia would lead one to believe. These persons reported that they were traumatized by much that they heard. They phrased this in various ways: "They talked about me as if I weren't there"; "they acted as if I didn't have any brains or feelings"; "they often sounded as though they thought I was as good as dead, and then of course I wanted to be."

There is a usual assumption that when a patient cannot or does not respond he does not receive. This inference may be unwarranted. Every patient interviewed indicated that his capacity to understand returned very shortly after his trauma and that it consistently increased long before he was able to respond to what he heard. Many stated that in the immediate post-trauma period they experienced fear and anguish. They believed these feelings might have been assuaged had they received reassurance and even some explanation of what had happened to them. But, as they commented to us, "nobody talked *to* me, only *about* me."

SPEED OF INPUT The aphasic persons all thought that they would have achieved successful communication earlier if the speakers had spoken more slowly. One patient compared the rate of speech he heard to the sound produced when a tape recorder is played at a high speed. One patient said that when conversation was too fast "it was just noise to me." Another was able to say, "I hear all right but, you see, I hear more slowly since my stroke."

AMOUNT OF INPUT The project participants all agreed that "everyone asks too many questions at one time." The person with aphasia is often unable to formulate a reply under optimal conditions. Any interfering stimulus, such as a second question or even a repetition of the first question, can prevent his processing an answer. Yet, under these conditions, the patient's progress is often judged by his responses. His chart may read as a result of this input overload, "Patient unable to answer questions." This entry may affect treatment planning and consequently the patient's entire future. Actually a barrage of questions can disrupt communication flow for a normal speaker. Parents, teachers, police, and lawyers frequently use it as a disruptive approach in certain situations. Our respondents assured us that, even early in their recovery period, they could have answered some questions presented to them if they had been asked one at a time.

LENGTH OF RESPONSE TIME The respondents said that they needed more time to prepare and produce an answer. Their general impression was that no one waited a sufficient length of time for an answer. Many reported frustration on numerous occasions by the interruption of their thoughts with repetition of questions just as they were about to reply. "When everybody tried to hurry me, all they did was throw sand in my gears" and "I think my wheels go round a great deal slower now, but nobody seems to know this but me."

PERCEPTION OF CUES The aphasic patients displayed awareness of and sensitivity to nonverbal communication from the personnel around them. It is of course true that many persons, including hospital personnel and family members, have difficulty tolerating the consequences of the aphasic persons' impairment. Most people control any overt indications of their annoyance at delayed or inappropriate responses. Yet they are frequently unaware that this behavior is inadequate. The participants cited numerous subtle signs of impatience from those around them which were deeply discouraging—audible sighs, tightening of the mouth muscles, shoulder and eye movements, and drumming fingers. The aphasic persons agreed that such behavior affected their morale, motivation, and progress adversely.

LEVEL OF EVALUATION TESTS The participants considered many of the tasks they were directed to perform during a test or treatment as silly, useless, or insultingly childish. They were particularly emphatic about requests to recite the alphabet; use of childish language, pictures, concepts, and stories; and tests and drills involving nonsense syllables. They objected to the uselessness of counting backwards and repeating numbers in reverse order. They were puzzled by the number of demands for information they thought the questioner already possessed. When several people in the same institution presented the same or almost the same test materials successively, the respondents concluded that the hospital either did not know what it was doing or cared so little that no one knew the test had already been performed.

Participants had been daunted by the testers' manner, which was either bellicose or indifferent. Questions were hurled at the aphasic person in a voice that somewhat frightened him or were presented so blandly as to extinguish motivation for cooperation. One patient said that a questioner "barked at me as if I were a dog. I thought he might hit me if I answered." The reverse effect obtained with another aphasic person: "I felt he couldn't care less and probably wouldn't listen even if I did say something."

In some disciplines, seemingly useless tasks may yield useful information. But if the patient does not understand this, he may fail to respond not because he *cannot* but because he *declines* to. He may be rejecting conduct he considers foolish in an adult.

DESTRUCTIVENESS OF NOISE Noise pollution and its effects were described in many ways: "I thought I was going noise crazy!" "I always thought a hospital was supposed to be a quiet place. It was worse than the airport."

The participants said that noise hurt them "and not just in the ear." They thought much of the noise was avoidable with a little care and some common-sense rules. All mentioned the prevalence of television sets, their high volume, and their continuous output. They suggested that earphones be required for all hospital sets. They also commented on the loud voices of hospital personnel and suggested that room doors be kept closed to contain noise. They also mentioned door slamming, pan rattling, loud bells, and constant loudspeaker announcements, as well as squealing wheels on hospital equipment.

Any high level of noise generated in a hospital is usually amplified by the hard wall and floors that are installed to facilitate cleaning. Noise studies in hospitals by an audiologist could identify sources of ambient sound that might be reduced.

INFLUX OF PERSONNEL In the participants' opinions, they were observed too frequently by too many varied groups. These unidentified people, whom the aphasic person did not see as related to his illness, appeared unexpectedly around his bed, in his physical therapy cubicle, or in the examining room. All participants reported that this invasion of their space irritated them seriously. One person said that after this experience he knew how the animals at the zoo felt on holidays.

The size of the groups was disturbing, too. When we explained that these were teaching visits, all the participants voiced their willingness to contribute to health education. They remarked, however, that had someone explained the visits to them before they were made, the visits would have been more tolerable. They suggested less frequent visits, smaller groups, and that lectures about a patient's medical condition be held elsewhere before the bedside visit.

NEED FOR INFORMATION Many decisions affecting patients are made for administrative or medical reasons—frequently, it seems to the patient, without considering his viewpoint. Aphasic persons see this as lack of regard for their feelings and even for their rights. They expressed a need to have explanations as well as directives and orders. The usual assumptions that aphasic persons do not understand and that consequently explanations are superfluous were both contradicted by this study.

RESPECT FOR PERSONHOOD Irrelevant questions which violate the aphasic person's privacy and often injure his dignity were mentioned. Those most frequently cited were inquiries concerning his finances. The manner and imputations rather than the basic inquiry were considered offensive.

The participants regarded their progress as a private matter and resented the frequent requests to "show off" their achievement.

RESPONSIVENESS TO NEEDS The last point the group made is common to every modern organization: "Too much yakketty before any action." The participants thought that responses to their needs and wants were needlessly delayed, a delay that was in some way related to their inability to talk.

The data from these aphasic patients cast additional light on two long-held tenets in aphasiology concerning spontaneous recovery and short duration of treatment.

The spontaneous recovery period is usually described as the six to twelve weeks immediately post-trauma. It has been assumed that the patient will recover language during this time. Yet from the data we obtained, this period would be better termed "optimum treatment period," the period when early speech rehabilitation is initiated.

The second insight concerned the duration of treatment. These patients demonstrated that additional improvement, sometimes at a very high level, can and does take place for two or more years following onset.

Consistent exploration of patient feedback in aphasia may provide a basis for further reevaluation of treatment policies and procedures. Such feedback may be important in modifying the behavior of those who care for the patients. The nurse is in a prime position to apply the feedback results to reduce patient frustration and accelerate speech rehabilitation.

Resocializing...Through a Stroke Club

HELEN M. FALKNOR • BEVERLY J. HARRIS

Stroke victims and their families can help.

As the two nurse coordinators of an RMP stroke project, we learned that stroke patients and their families had many unmet needs and concerns, even though they had excellent follow-up from local home health agencies. In collecting data about stroke patients, particularly in the post-acute phase, we frequently were told that a patient wouldn't leave his house. "He's too embarrassed to go out in public" was a common report, because of residual disability from the stroke. And just as often, we were asked how patients with similar difficulties handled the problem. "If we could just get together with families with similar problems, I know Dave can't be the only one with these feelings."

We shared our findings with the stroke team at one of four acute care hospitals in our county. Our task was not only to collect data on all stroke patients in the county but also to provide continuity of care by encouraging a team approach to care in each hospital and extended care facility in our area. The hospital team recognized the value of a stroke club and began work on its creation.

SECURING SERVICES

The first thing the group did was to appoint an advisory board made up of interested lay and professional people in the community. This

---

MRS. FALKNOR (B.S.N. and M.S., University of California School of Nursing, San Francisco) is a nursing consultant with the State of California Department of Health. She formerly was coordinator in the stroke project described here. MRS. HARRIS (B.S., California State University, San Jose) is the nurse coordinator of the Santa Cruz County Regional Medical Program Stroke Project, which was funded by the California RMP, Area III, Stanford University School of Medicine, Palo Alto, Calif.

board has since proven to be instrumental in securing a meeting place, getting publicity in the newspapers, arranging for transportation to the club meetings for members who cannot drive, and getting informational brochures printed about the club. Many of these services were secured through existing community resources.

Following the planning meetings, we (the nurse coordinators) contacted a group of potential stroke club participants and invited them to a meeting. The selection was arbitrary: we contacted those individuals whom we recognized as having leadership abilities, an interest in such a group, and the motivation to function actively in making the club a success.

The local visiting nurse association offered its conference room for the meeting and, on a rainy afternoon in November, the club met for the first time with a total of 25 people—stroke victims and spouses. A physical therapist who had worked with several of these patients and was skilled in group process was selected as guest speaker.

With her help, we were able to provide an environment for the group to begin to explore the future direction of the club, to become acquainted with each other, and to realize the club's potential in solving some of their problems. The opportunity to share ideas in a physically and emotionally comfortable setting proved to be an essential factor in getting the club started.

The charter members decided that the purpose of the club should be: to provide educational assistance to stroke patients and their families and to offer a supportive milieu that would help them in the difficult task of resocialization.

SETTING PRIORITIES

During the first few meetings, the group concentrated on the organizational and decision-making process necessary for the growth of a club. A slate of officers was elected, bylaws were developed and approved, and committee chairmen were appointed. The club members decided not to differentiate between patients and spouses; both could vote and hold office. The elected president and vice-president were stroke victims, while the secretary and treasurer were spouses.

The club members also voted against dues but decided to establish an informal plan for coffee donations. They were afraid that a required fee of any amount would make membership prohibitive for some stroke patients. A schedule of monthly mid-afternoon meetings was agreed upon as the most convenient times for the majority of members.

For many stroke patients, attendance at the monthly club meeting has been the only out-of-the-house contact or activity they had had since their stroke. From the beginning, we were careful in our roles as nurse coordinators not to dominate the group. At first, the group tended to look to us for leadership and guidance, and we sometimes had difficulty in deciding when to provide leadership and when to stand back and let the leadership emerge from the group. But we constantly assessed the group's progress and supported and encouraged the member's independence. We felt strongly that the stroke club must be the *members'* organization and acted primarily as consultants to assure that the decision-making process would be in their hands.

During the early months, we contacted speakers, brought refreshments, arranged for transportation, and provided secretarial services. As the club members became more involved in the group they elected committees to be responsible for these activities. At the same time, we gradually but steadily withdrew from an active role in the club's organization. For example, a committee was formed to locate a permanent meeting place, and each potential site was visited by three committee members who then reported their findings to the group.

We offered assistance when it was requested by the committee, but we did not participate in the final decision. Eventually, a multi-purpose room in an elementary school was secured at no cost to the group. This activity provided a framework for the patients to begin to feel like useful human beings again, capable of making choices and helping each other with common problems.

The guest speakers provided one form of education. In addition, the club members educated each other by sharing experiences and encouraging each other to try to do things they thought were impossible. The coffee hour following the formal meeting became an important time for members to engage in this sharing process. The significance of this kind of empathic interaction was summed up by a patient who said, "It means so much more to hear encouragement and suggestions from another stroke patient than it does if they come from someone like a nurse or social workers." Friendships have been established that continue outside of club meetings; some people telephone each other frequently, others provide transportation for new friends who do not drive.

The fact that this group has become viable in less than a year is particularly significant, since the average age of the club members is seventy. Due to psychosocial and health factors, the older person in our society, even without disability from strokes, is frequently more reluctant to respond or become actively committed to outreach programs. However, if a program such as ours provides the older person with a sense of his importance and identity in a group he will more easily develop a feeling of trust and security in himself and with others.

The membership has a variety of disabilities, ranging from no noticeable impairment to those requiring wheelchairs. Many have severe communication problems. There is also a broad spectrum of socioeconomic and educational levels. The group is primarily white, which has prompted the members to think about developing an outreach program to attract more stroke victims from minority groups. Seventy percent of the stroke victims in the club are male, and 58 percent are married. Most of the spouses also attend meetings. Only three members live in nursing homes, and two reside in boarding homes.

EXPANDING ACTIVITIES

In the spring of 1972, the advisory board met again and four club members attended as guests. Their contribution led to a more active and involved advisory board and to the decision that the club should become the Stroke Information Center for the county. A central telephone line was secured so that anyone who desired information about the club, stroke care, community resources, and so forth could phone the number. The calls were handled by volunteers from the club or by us.

The club members have also developed a protocol to contact stroke victims while they are still in the hospital to inform them about the club. Either a club member or a volunteer uses this initial contact to assume the role of advocate for the patient and his family, visiting him at home and escorting him to club meetings. As a result, a training program is being developed based on specific information about the causes, treatment, and problems associated with stroke in order to prepare members to work effectively with stroke patients. Thus, the member will have not only his own personal experiences but also this additional knowledge to draw upon as he tries to meet new stroke victims' needs.

A speakers bureau has been established to recruit therapists, social workers, physicians, and other health personnel who are willing to talk with the group at monthly meetings. The therapists have been particularly well received, indicating that many of the club's members have numerous concerns and questions that have not been satisfactorily dealt with during the acute phase of their illness. For many, this is the only opportunity to obtain help with some of their problems. At one meeting, for instance, a speech pathologist was confronting various couples with some of the feelings they had been unable to express previously. When a wife said that her husband used to be an intelligent man, the speech pathologist retorted with, "What do you mean he *used* to be intelligent?"

Although such a frank open discussion could lead to disastrous consequences, the feedback from this meeting was astounding—a unanimous, "The best one we've ever had."

HIDDEN ADVANTAGES

It is difficult to evaluate the dynamics of group interaction in the club, because of its very nature. In reducing human behavior to data, the risk of destroying the meaning of the behavior is great. However, we do see certain gains. The rapid growth in membership from 25 to 100 within two years suggests that the club is meeting some needs of many stroke patients and their spouses. The informative talks given at the request of the club members by a wide representation from the health team points to the members' search for knowledge to better deal with problems that result from stroke.

Yet how do we deal with factors that do not lend themselves to coding and analysis? For example, how can we know the significance of daily telephone calls to check on the safety and needs of another less fortunate stroke victim, or measure the benefits of picnics and potluck dinners that are the sole social activities for many members? We do see, however, an increase in the club's activities. An outreach program is being formed and efforts are being made to draw more nursing home patients into the club. Also, the members plan to relay more information about stroke—its causes, prevention, and treatment—to the public. At the same time, they hope to make the community more aware of the needs of stroke patients and to seek the public's support for stroke programs.

The stroke club, although still in an early stage, has already demonstrated to its members that illness and permanent disability need not mean the loss of a useful life.

Autumn Months, Autumn Years

MARION B. DOLAN

The patient had had a stroke and her husband was legally blind, yet with this nurse's help they became a couple again.

After the first four months of our independent nursing practice, it became more feasible to divide the patients according to travel time and distance from our office. As a result, it was I who drove out to meet our newest patient, Ms. A., one crisp September morning.

From the history we had received from her son, I learned that she was totally bedridden. She had had a CVA which affected her left side and then a fracture of the right femur. As I drove, I mused that probably the one person I enjoyed working with least was the elderly woman with an orthopedic condition. I knew I had to overcome this feeling before taking care of Ms. A.

We had spent quite a while explaining to her son that we made only house calls and could not stay a full eight hours. The family had requested private duty nurses for the day and evening. Since the registry had no one available, we agreed to make two house calls daily until a private duty nurse was available.

The A.'s ranch-style house, situated on a lovely piece of property, surrounded by many low shrubs, flowers, and stately trees, seemed ideal for an elderly couple.

Mr. A greeted me at the door. He looked much older than I had anticipated. I'd been told that Ms. A. was 73 and I had no way of knowing that Mr. A. was 10 years older. He had a broad smile and I realized as he welcomed me that he was totally blind. He immediately led me to his

---

MS. DOLAN, *R.N., is director of nursing, Maple Leaf Health Care Facility, Manchester, N.H. She was a part-time independent practitioner when the article was written.*

wife's room and announced expansively, "Here's Betty" It was as though he were introducing a smash Broadway hit. Once he had assured me I'd find everything I'd need in the "sickroom" or the bathroom, he left me alone with Ms. A.

Ms. A. had an aura of classic beauty. Her sheets, instead of being stark white, bore a bright floral pattern. The dresser held an array of cosmetics. Over her hospital bed, a makeshift shelf was stacked with Chux, back-rub lotion, and other supplies. There was also a strong odor of feces.

I introduced myself to Ms. A., but received no response. Was she deaf? Did she have a receptive or expressive aphasia? I longed for the security of a chart or Kardex. Until this time all our patients had had a family member at home who could give a complete, reliable history. Ms. A.'s son had given me only a list of four doctors who had been caring for her. I would bathe her and call one of them. Mr. A., I thought, wouldn't be an accurate historian—a wrong judgment as I soon learned.

I began by explaining that I would start her bath by removing the soiled sheet. It's much pleasanter for an incontinent person if I remove the source of an offending odor before doing anything else. Then she can enjoy her bath, and it's more therapeutic and relaxing. As I rolled Ms. A. over on her side, she was staring out the window without any expression.

"It must be very difficult for you not to have any control over your bodily functions."

She turned her head slowly and said, "You are the first person who has realized that I don't go in the bed on purpose."

I explained that often after a patient has had a stroke she is unable to control her voiding or bowel movements. I was overjoyed that Ms. A. could hear and speak.

Walking down the hall to dispose of the soiled linen, I met Mr. A. He was upset that I might have finished her bath. I explained what I was doing, but he still seemed suspicious. I asked him when Ms. A. usually had bowel movements before she became ill.

"Like clockwork—always right after breakfast!"

I told him there was no reason we couldn't get her back to the same pattern. Other nurses had tried the commode, he said, but "the darn thing didn't work." I suggested that if she had a suppository before breakfast this might stimulate her to have a bowel movement. He promised to delay her breakfast until I arrived the next day, but he looked skeptical.

After I had finished her bath and changed the bed, I made the following nursing assessments: Ms. A. was incontinent of feces and urine, had a sacral decubitus ulcer, a paralyzed left arm, and could not walk. I called the family physician, who gave me an order for glycerine suppositories and wished me luck. He agreed that she could get out of bed provided she did not put weight on her right leg.

When I asked Mr. A. if he could obtain a wheelchair, he led me to a second bedroom which contained a commode, a huge box of Chux, and a wheelchair. With a note of sadness he said, "This is where Betty and I used to sleep." Now he slept on a day bed in Ms. A.'s "sickroom" so that he might help her during the night. I arranged to come back at 7:00 P.M. to prepare her for sleep and assured him I'd come at any other time I was needed. I had learned that Mr. A. was legally blind but still had 15 percent vision.

Just as I was leaving, Mr. A. said, "Nurse, might I ask your professional advice on something else?" I was ready with all kinds of intelligent, professional answers when he inquired seriously, "How long do you cook a chicken? Four hours at 400?"

Laughing, I told him I didn't think any chicken could take that. After looking at the chicken, I assured him that two hours at 325 degrees would be plenty. As I walked down the driveway, I realized that the A.'s most imperative need was to become as independent as possible in all their daily activities.

That evening, I got Ms. A. refreshed and into a wheelchair to watch television with her husband. After the program, I spoke to them about Ms. A.'s decubitus ulcer, explaining that it would never heal if she continued to sleep on it. Mr. A. said that until this illness Ms. A. had always slept on her abdomen. I reassured them that there was no reason Ms. A. couldn't resume her previous pattern. Mr. A. quickly pointed out that the sore hadn't healed in six months, that only a small scab had formed on one side. He was astonished when I said that the doctor could remove the scab to give the tissue under it a chance to heal.

From that night on, Ms. A. slept on her abdomen. I have often wondered why nurses avoid placing patients in the prone position. The usual hospital patient lies on his back in semi-Fowler's position, his arms neatly at his side, covers tightly tucked in at his feet. I have long since decided that a sloppy bed is a sign of good nursing care.

I left to meet my associate for our nightly discussion of the day's activities. We often glean valuable information from each other and, thus, a broader view of each patient. We cover for each other on our days off, so daily progress reports are essential. She agreed with my preliminary plans and suggested asking the doctor for a follow-up x-ray to determine whether Ms. A.'s fracture had healed. If so, we could begin walker training.

The next morning I gave Ms. A. a glycerine suppository, then helped her transfer to her commode for breakfast. Twenty minutes after her meal, Ms. A. had a large bowel movement. Mr. A. looked at me in awe even though I had explained that the body would resume old habits with little help.

I started a 15-minute passive range-of-motion exercise to her affected limbs. Mr. A. was interested in what I was doing, so I asked him to do the same exercises twice in the afternoon. I would then do them once more at night. He learned quickly and showed great patience. I explained that the exercises would strengthen the muscles that weren't being used. Ms. A. would be able to use them when she started walking. Even though our bowel training program had started off successfully, Mr. A. couldn't believe that his wife might soon be able to walk.

After the first week I called their family physician to relate Ms. A.'s progress. He scheduled an x-ray and debridement of the ulcer for the following week. Mr. A. and I arranged for transportation with the town's emergency squad.

Our trip to the hospital proved rewarding. Mr. and Ms. A. were delighted with the orthopedic surgeon's news that Ms. A.'s right femur was now ready for full weight bearing. Until this time she had been pivoting to her wheelchair or commode. Her walker would give her the freedom to use the bathroom after breakfast. We had been unable to do this because the bathroom doorway was too narrow for her wheelchair.

The walker training took several weeks and it was not without problems. I had never realized how difficult it is to use a walker on a carpeted floor. The patient must remember to lift the walker a little higher when moving it. To help overcome "carpet drag," Ms. A. changed to leather-soled shoes which did not hold her back as her rubber-soled slippers had done.

After I'd been seeing the A.'s for several weeks, I realized fall was beginning its annual display of color, that each morning was a little crisper. As I arrived one day, smoke from a delightful, crackling fire was rising from the chimney. The open fire proved a tremendous boost to Ms. A.'s spirits. She loved to watch it and feel its warmth. From the middle of October, there was always a fire to look forward to.

Although I tried to help Ms. A. void regularly, her incontinence could not be solved because she had a neurogenic bladder. She began to wear toddler-sized Pampers and adult rubber pants. I bathed her in the morning and then she sat in the living room to watch television or the fire until I returned in the evening. With her husband's help, she did push-ups in the chair to relieve pressure on her buttocks.

Her bath pattern had changed, too. She now washed her face and hands at the sink and I finished her bath. She brushed her dentures after they had been soaked. The first morning I had Ms. A. perform these tasks herself, Mr. A. commented later that they were paying me well to do these things for her. I explained that, like the bowel and walker training, it was my job to teach Ms. A. to be as self-sufficient as possible. The next day I added hair brushing and combing to her activities.

From the day I met Ms. A., I used some of her perfume or toilet water with her bath. There were seven bottles when we started. Ms. A. asked me when she'd be better. I told her that she would never be as she was before her illness but, by the time we'd used up all the perfume, she'd be so independent that I would not be needed. It was a peculiar goal to set. As we began to empty the bottles, we would also measure her progress. She continued to do well.

I had been manicuring Ms. A.'s nails once a week. This helped me to see that doing one patient's nails can be as therapeutic for her as a back rub is for someone else. She had never asked me to do them, but was more than pleased when I offered.

I also began teaching Mr. A. how to care for her. I showed him our bath routine. He was able to walk with her when she used the walker. Slowly the A.'s were becoming independent.

At night I found them side by side, holding hands and watching TV. There seemed to be no reason why Ms. A. must continue sleeping in the hospital bed in the sickroom. I thought about a sexuality course I had taken and how important it is for the elderly to live like normal men and women. The A.'s needed the full companionship they had always shared.

When I proposed the change, they were overjoyed. I helped Mr. A. put the bedroom back as it had been. We moved all leftover supplies into the sickroom so that their bedroom had no aura of illness. The double bed was next to a wall and I suggested that Ms. A. sleep on that side for safety. They informed me that was her side anyway. I jokingly replied, "You've been protecting her for quite a while."

"Yes," he stated proudly, "for 61 years."

The two of them no longer needed me at night so we cancelled those visits. The next morning we decided that we could also cancel the day visits.

It was Thanksgiving week and saying good-bye was difficult. The A.'s son and daughter-in-law were coming for dinner. As I was leaving, Mr. A. asked one more "professional" question—"How long should I cook my turkey—eight hours at 400?" After I told him what temperature to use, he pointed to a blackboard. Originally it had displayed two telephone numbers in 18-inch numerals—his son's and the doctor's. Now there were three numbers; ours was at the top of the list because he said "sometimes my son's at work but you're always available." Tears stung my eyes as I walked down the driveway. We had accomplished our goal of rehabilitation.

As I drove to my next patient, I realized that the leaves had nearly finished falling. The young trees, it seemed to me, had lost their beautiful hues first. The older trees were struggling to keep theirs, almost defiantly, against the first blows of winter. As the elm and oak cling tenaciously to their foliage, so the elderly make a valiant effort to hold on to their dignity and independence.

When my associate and I discussed the patients we had seen that day, I paused at the A.'s chart. How do you sum up all the human things that had happened? Her decubitus had healed. She could walk with the assistive walker. She was bowel trained. Those were the facts! I wanted to include the anecdotes about the chicken and the turkey and, finally, to mention that there were still one-and-a-half bottles of perfume left.

I made follow-up telephone calls and was delighted to learn that the A.'s had no further problems. There is great satisfaction in seeing how patients can grow with up-to-date nursing care based on nursing assessment and goals.